# Caregiver Log Book

_____
Name of Patient / Client

_____
Date of Birth

From _____
Month/Day/Year

To _____
Month/Day/Year

Is there a DNR (Do Not Resuscitate) on File?
If yes, LOCATION of DNR:

Copyright 2015 Karen Delaporte
www.amazon.com

# Contact Information

| | NAME | PHONE | ADDRESS |
|---|---|---|---|
| ICE - In Case of Emergency | | | |
| Power of Med Attorney | | | |
| Spouse | | | |
| Daughter | | | |
| Son | | | |
| Grandchild | | | |
| Other Family | | | |
| Primary Dr. | | | |
| Cardiologist | | | |
| Chiropractor | | | |
| Gynecologist | | | |
| Naturopath | | | |
| Neurologist | | | |
| Oncologist | | | |
| Psychiatrist | | | |
| Rheumatologist | | | |
| Other Doctor | | | |
| Grocery Store | | | |

"Can I help you?" "No. I just waited 30 minutes to say 'Hi'." folksdaily.com

# Contact Information

| | NAME | PHONE | ADDRESS |
|---|---|---|---|
| Drugstore | | | |
| Medical Clinic | | | |
| Occupational Therapist | | | |
| Pharmacy | | | |
| Physical Therapist | | | |
| Post Office | | | |
| Speech Therapist | | | |
| Transportation | | | |
| Visiting Nurse | | | |
| Caregiver | | | |
| Caregiver | | | |
| Caregiver | | | |
| Caregiver | | | |
| Caregiver | | | |
| Caregiver | | | |
| | | | |
| | | | |

**My Phone Number:** 

"Grandchildren are not just for loving; they are for helping too."
Olivia (7 yrs. old) - Submitted by Gabrielle Childe --- U.K.

| ALLERGIES | CHRONIC MEDICAL CONDITIONS |
|---|---|
| **Prescriptions:** | |
| Chemical Sensitivities: | |
| Animals: | |
| Pollen: | |
| Flowers / Grasses / Mold: | |

"Life never seems to be the way we want it, but we live it the best way we can. There is no perfect life, but we can fill it with perfect moments." 2007 Farzana Siddiqui

# CAREGIVER SCHEDULE

**YEAR** _____   **MONTH** _____

| SUNDAY | MONDAY | TUESDAY | WEDNESDAY | THURSDAY | FRIDAY | SATURDAY |
|--------|--------|---------|-----------|----------|--------|----------|
|        |        |         |           |          |        |          |
|        |        |         |           |          |        |          |
|        |        |         |           |          |        |          |
|        |        |         |           |          |        |          |
|        |        |         |           |          |        |          |

## TEN FACTS ABOUT YOU

1. You're reading this right now.
2. You're realizing that is a stupid fact.
4. You didn't realize I skipped three.
5. You're checking now.
6. You're smiling.
7. You're still reading this even tho it's stupid.
9. You didn't realize I skipped eight.
10. You're checking again & can't believe you fell for it again.
11. You're enjoying this.
12. You didn't realize there's only supposed to be ten.

findmemes.com

YOU! Yes, You!
The one reading this.
You are beautiful, talented, amazing, and simply the best at being you!
NEVER FORGET THAT.

# CAREGIVER SCHEDULE

**MONTH** _____  
**YEAR** _____

| SUNDAY | MONDAY | TUESDAY | WEDNESDAY | THURSDAY | FRIDAY | SATURDAY |
|--------|--------|---------|-----------|----------|--------|----------|
|        |        |         |           |          |        |          |
|        |        |         |           |          |        |          |
|        |        |         |           |          |        |          |
|        |        |         |           |          |        |          |
|        |        |         |           |          |        |          |

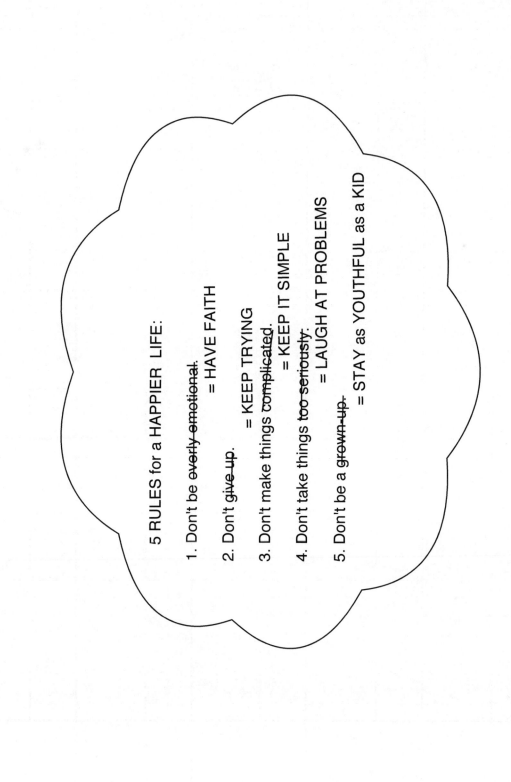

# CAREGIVER SCHEDULE

**MONTH** _____  **YEAR** _____

| SUNDAY | MONDAY | TUESDAY | WEDNESDAY | THURSDAY | FRIDAY | SATURDAY |
|--------|--------|---------|-----------|----------|--------|----------|
|        |        |         |           |          |        |          |
|        |        |         |           |          |        |          |
|        |        |         |           |          |        |          |
|        |        |         |           |          |        |          |
|        |        |         |           |          |        |          |

"Come into the kingdom prepared for you. For I was hungry, and you gave me something to eat; I was thirsty and you gave me something to drink; I was a stranger, and you invited me in; I needed clothes and you clothed me; I was sick and you took care of me; I was in prison and you visited me. Whatever you did for even one of the least of these, you did it for me." Jesus (Matthew 25:34-40)

# DAILY ROUTINE / SCHEDULE

| AM | Monday | Tuesday | Wednesday | Thursday | Friday | Saturday | Sunday |
|---|---|---|---|---|---|---|---|
| 5:00 | | | | | | | |
| 6:00 | | | | | | | |
| 7:00 | | | | | | | |
| 8:00 | | | | | | | |
| 9:00 | | | | | | | |
| 10:00 | | | | | | | |
| 11:00 | | | | | | | |
| NOON | | | | | | | |
| 1:00 PM | | | | | | | |
| 2:00 | | | | | | | |
| 3:00 | | | | | | | |
| 4:00 | | | | | | | |
| 5:00 | | | | | | | |
| 6:00 | | | | | | | |
| 7:00 | | | | | | | |
| 8:00 | | | | | | | |
| 9:00 | | | | | | | |
| 10:00 | | | | | | | |
| 11:00 | | | | | | | |
| AM | Monday | Tuesday | Wednesday | Thursday | Friday | Saturday | Sunday |

# CAREGIVER INSTRUCTIONS

**WAKE-UP ROUTINE:**

**BATH/SHOWER HAIRWASH:**

**BREAKFAST ROUTINE:**

**LUNCH ROUTINE:**

*"Kind words can be short and easy to speak, but their echoes are truly endless."* Mother Teresa

# CAREGIVER INSTRUCTIONS

**LEAVING-HOME ROUTINE:**

**TOILETING ROUTINE:**

**DINNERTIME ROUTINE:**

**BEDTIME ROUTINE:**

*"Early to bed, and early to rise, makes a man healthy, wealthy, and wise." Benjamin Franklin*

# Prescription Information

| Brand Name | Generic Name | Dosage | Doctor | Pharmacy |
|---|---|---|---|---|
| | | | | |
| | | | | |
| | | | | |
| | | | | |
| | | | | |
| | | | | |
| | | | | |
| | | | | |
| | | | | |
| | | | | |

*"Most of the important things in the world have been accomplished by people who kept on trying when there seemed to be no hope at all."* Dale Carnegie

# Prescription Information

| Brand Name | Generic Name | Dosage | Doctor | Pharmacy |
|---|---|---|---|---|
| | | | | |
| | | | | |
| | | | | |
| | | | | |
| | | | | |
| | | | | |
| | | | | |
| | | | | |
| | | | | |
| | | | | |

Location in home prescriptions are kept:

*"Treat everyone with kindness and respect. even those who are rude - not because they are nice - but because you are."*

# Supplement Information

| Supplement | Brand Name | Dosage | Misc Info | Store |
|---|---|---|---|---|
|  |  |  |  |  |
|  |  |  |  |  |
|  |  |  |  |  |
|  |  |  |  |  |
|  |  |  |  |  |
|  |  |  |  |  |
|  |  |  |  |  |
|  |  |  |  |  |
|  |  |  |  |  |
|  |  |  |  |  |

Location Supplements are kept:

"*Tears are prayers too, They travel to God when we can't speak.*" Psalm 56:8

# Medications/Supplements Schedule

| AM Medications | Dosage amt. | Lunch Medications | Dosage amt. | PM Medications | Dosage amt. |
|---|---|---|---|---|---|
|  |  |  |  |  |  |
|  |  |  |  |  |  |
|  |  |  |  |  |  |
|  |  |  |  |  |  |
|  |  |  |  |  |  |
|  |  |  |  |  |  |
|  |  |  |  |  |  |

Notes:

*"In this life, we cannot always do great things. But we can do small things with great love."*
*Mother Teresa*

# Activities My Client Enjoys

Favorite TV Station:

Favorite TV News Station:

Favorite TV Shows / Time:

Favorite Movies:

Things he/she enjoys talking about:

Puzzles - Number Pieces:

Card Games:

Board Games:

Outdoor Activities:

Places I Like to Go:

Magazines:

Newspaper:

Pets Names:

Children's Names:

Grandchildren's Names:

Great-Grandchildren's Names:

*"We should keep on encouraging each other to be thoughtful, & to do do helpful things."* Heb. 10:24

# Foods/Drinks My Client Enjoys

|  |  |
|---|---|
|  |  |
|  |  |
|  |  |
|  |  |
|  |  |
|  |  |
|  |  |
|  |  |
|  |  |
|  |  |

| Food Allergies/Sensitivities: | Foods to Avoid or do NOT like: |
|---|---|
|  |  |

| DATE: | | | DAY OF WEEK: | | | | | | |
|---|---|---|---|---|---|---|---|---|---|
| TIME | | | | ORAL INTAKE | | | | OUTPUT | |
| | am | pm | Caregiver | Medications / Supplements | Dosage amt. | Food | Liquid | Urine | BM |
| | | | | | | | | | |
| | | | | | | | | | |
| | | | | | | | | | |
| | | | | | | | | | |
| | | | | | | | | | |
| | | | | | | | | | |

Notes:

*"Let your faith be bigger than your fear."* www.quotesgram.com

| HYGIENE Teeth/Bathe Hair/Nails | Physical Therapy | Occupational Therapy | Speech Therapy | Sleep | Vitals Y/N on chart | P/M Index |
|---|---|---|---|---|---|---|
| | | | | | | |
| | | | | | | |
| | | | | | | |
| | | | | | | |
| | | | | | | |
| | | | | | | |

Notes:

PAIN / MOOD
Index
0-10
0=none/good
10=high/angry

| DATE: | | | | DAY OF WEEK: | | | | |
|---|---|---|---|---|---|---|---|---|
| TIME | | | | ORAL INTAKE | | | OUTPUT | |
| | am | pm | Caregiver | Medications / Supplements | Dosage amt. | Food | Liquid | Urine | BM |
| | | | | | | | | | |
| | | | | | | | | | |
| | | | | | | | | | |
| | | | | | | | | | |
| | | | | | | | | | |
| | | | | | | | | | |

Notes:

*"Instead of living in the shadows of yesterday, live in the light of today, and the hope of tomorrow."*
*www.quotesgram.com*

| HYGIENE Teeth/Bathe Hair/Nails | Physical Therapy | Occupational Therapy | Speech Therapy | Sleep | Vitals Y/N on chart | P/M Index |
|---|---|---|---|---|---|---|
|  |  |  |  |  |  |  |
|  |  |  |  |  |  |  |
|  |  |  |  |  |  |  |
|  |  |  |  |  |  |  |
|  |  |  |  |  |  |  |
|  |  |  |  |  |  |  |

Notes:

PAIN / MOOD
Index
0-10
0=none/good
10=high/angry

| DATE: | | | | DAY OF WEEK: | | | | |
|---|---|---|---|---|---|---|---|---|
| TIME | | | | ORAL INTAKE | | | OUTPUT | |
| | am | pm | Caregiver | Medications / Supplements | Dosage amt. | Food | Liquid | Urine | BM |
| | | | | | | | | | |
| | | | | | | | | | |
| | | | | | | | | | |
| | | | | | | | | | |
| | | | | | | | | | |
| | | | | | | | | | |

Notes:

*"You will learn a lot about yourself if you stretch in the direction of goodness, of bigness, of kindness, of forgiveness, of emotional bravery. Be a warrior for love.*
*Cheryl Strayed thechristianleftblog.org*

| HYGIENE Teeth/Bathe Hair/Nails | Physical Therapy | Occupational Therapy | Speech Therapy | Sleep | Vitals Y/N on chart | P/M Index |
|---|---|---|---|---|---|---|
| | | | | | | |
| | | | | | | |
| | | | | | | |
| | | | | | | |
| | | | | | | |
| | | | | | | |

Notes:

PAIN / MOOD
Index
0-10
0=none/good
10=high/angry

| DATE: | | | | DAY OF WEEK: | | | | |
|---|---|---|---|---|---|---|---|---|
| TIME | | | | ORAL INTAKE | | | OUTPUT | |
| | am | pm | Caregiver | Medications / Supplements | Dosage amt. | Food | Liquid | Urine | BM |
| | | | | | | | | | |
| | | | | | | | | | |
| | | | | | | | | | |
| | | | | | | | | | |
| | | | | | | | | | |
| | | | | | | | | | |

Notes:

*"Small acts, when multiplied by millions of people, can transform the world."* quotesgram.com

| HYGIENE Teeth/Bathe Hair/Nails | Physical Therapy | Occupational Therapy | Speech Therapy | Sleep | Vitals Y/N on chart | P/M Index |
|---|---|---|---|---|---|---|
| | | | | | | |
| | | | | | | |
| | | | | | | |
| | | | | | | |
| | | | | | | |
| | | | | | | |

Notes:

PAIN / MOOD
Index
0-10
0=none/good
10=high/angry

| DATE: | | | | DAY OF WEEK: | | | | | |
|---|---|---|---|---|---|---|---|---|---|
| TIME | | | | ORAL INTAKE | | | | OUTPUT | |
| | am | pm | Caregiver | Medications / Supplements | Dosage amt. | Food | Liquid | Urine | BM |
| | | | | | | | | | |
| | | | | | | | | | |
| | | | | | | | | | |
| | | | | | | | | | |
| | | | | | | | | | |
| | | | | | | | | | |

Notes:

*"Kindness is a language the deaf can hear and the blind can see." Mark Twain*

| HYGIENE Teeth/Bathe Hair/Nails | Physical Therapy | Occupational Therapy | Speech Therapy | Sleep | Vitals Y/N on chart | P/M Index |
|---|---|---|---|---|---|---|
| | | | | | | |
| | | | | | | |
| | | | | | | |
| | | | | | | |
| | | | | | | |
| | | | | | | |

Notes:

PAIN / MOOD
Index
0-10
0=none/good
10=high/angry

| DATE: | | | | DAY OF WEEK: | | | |
|---|---|---|---|---|---|---|---|
| TIME | | Caregiver | ORAL INTAKE |||| OUTPUT ||
| am | pm | | Medications / Supplements | Dosage amt. | Food | Liquid | Urine | BM |
| | | | | | | | | |
| | | | | | | | | |
| | | | | | | | | |
| | | | | | | | | |
| | | | | | | | | |
| | | | | | | | | |

NOTES:

*"Three essentials to happiness are something to do, someone to love, and something to hope for."*

| HYGIENE Teeth/Bathe Hair/Nails | Physical Therapy | Occupational Therapy | Speech Therapy | Sleep | Vitals Y/N on chart | P/M Index |
|---|---|---|---|---|---|---|
| | | | | | | |
| | | | | | | |
| | | | | | | |
| | | | | | | |
| | | | | | | |
| | | | | | | |

Notes:

PAIN / MOOD
Index
0-10
0=none/good
10=high/angry

| DATE: | | | | DAY OF WEEK: | | | | |
|---|---|---|---|---|---|---|---|---|
| TIME | | | | ORAL INTAKE | | | OUTPUT | |
| | am | pm | Caregiver | Medications / Supplements | Dosage amt. | Food | Liquid | Urine | BM |
| | | | | | | | | | |
| | | | | | | | | | |
| | | | | | | | | | |
| | | | | | | | | | |
| | | | | | | | | | |
| | | | | | | | | | |

Notes:

*"If we believe that tomorrow will be better, we can bear hardship today."*
*Thich Nhat Hanh quotesgram.com*

| HYGIENE Teeth/Bathe Hair/Nails | Physical Therapy | Occupational Therapy | Speech Therapy | Sleep | Vitals Y/N on chart | P/M Index |
|---|---|---|---|---|---|---|
| | | | | | | |
| | | | | | | |
| | | | | | | |
| | | | | | | |
| | | | | | | |
| | | | | | | |

Notes:

PAIN / MOOD Index
0-10
0=none/good
10=high/angry

| DATE: | | | | DAY OF WEEK: | | | | | |
|---|---|---|---|---|---|---|---|---|---|
| TIME | | | | ORAL INTAKE | | | | OUTPUT | |
| | am | pm | Caregiver | Medications / Supplements | Dosage amt. | Food | Liquid | Urine | BM |
| | | | | | | | | | |
| | | | | | | | | | |
| | | | | | | | | | |
| | | | | | | | | | |
| | | | | | | | | | |
| | | | | | | | | | |

Notes:

*"We are wise if while we wait for God to change our situation, we allow Him to change our hearts."*
*Karen Delaporte*

| HYGIENE Teeth/Bathe Hair/Nails | Physical Therapy | Occupational Therapy | Speech Therapy | Sleep | Vitals Y/N on chart | P/M Index |
|---|---|---|---|---|---|---|
|  |  |  |  |  |  |  |
|  |  |  |  |  |  |  |
|  |  |  |  |  |  |  |
|  |  |  |  |  |  |  |
|  |  |  |  |  |  |  |
|  |  |  |  |  |  |  |

Notes:

PAIN / MOOD
Index
0-10
0=none/good
10=high/angry

| DATE: | | | | DAY OF WEEK: | | | | |
|---|---|---|---|---|---|---|---|---|
| TIME | | | | ORAL INTAKE | | | OUTPUT | |
| | am | pm | Caregiver | Medications / Supplements | Dosage amt. | Food | Liquid | Urine | BM |
| | | | | | | | | | |
| | | | | | | | | | |
| | | | | | | | | | |
| | | | | | | | | | |
| | | | | | | | | | |
| | | | | | | | | | |
| | | | | | | | | | |

**Notes:**

*"When you find yourself cocooned in isolation and despair, and cannot find your way out of the darkness; remember, this is similar to the place where caterpillars go to grow their wings."*
*Calming your Inner Storm*

| HYGIENE Teeth/Bathe Hair/Nails | Physical Therapy | Occupational Therapy | Speech Therapy | Sleep | Vitals Y/N on chart | P/M Index |
|---|---|---|---|---|---|---|
|  |  |  |  |  |  |  |
|  |  |  |  |  |  |  |
|  |  |  |  |  |  |  |
|  |  |  |  |  |  |  |
|  |  |  |  |  |  |  |
|  |  |  |  |  |  |  |

Notes:

PAIN / MOOD
Index
0-10
0=none/good
10=high/angry

| DATE: | | | | DAY OF WEEK: | | | | |
|---|---|---|---|---|---|---|---|---|
| TIME | | | | ORAL INTAKE | | | OUTPUT | |
| | am | pm | Caregiver | Medications / Supplements | Dosage amt. | Food | Liquid | Urine | BM |
| | | | | | | | | | |
| | | | | | | | | | |
| | | | | | | | | | |
| | | | | | | | | | |
| | | | | | | | | | |
| | | | | | | | | | |

**Notes:**

*"Just when the caterpillar thought the world was over, it became a butterfly."*

| HYGIENE Teeth/Bathe Hair/Nails | Physical Therapy | Occupational Therapy | Speech Therapy | Sleep | Vitals Y/N on chart | P/M Index |
|---|---|---|---|---|---|---|
| | | | | | | |
| | | | | | | |
| | | | | | | |
| | | | | | | |
| | | | | | | |
| | | | | | | |

Notes:

PAIN / MOOD
Index
0-10
0=none/good
10=high/angry

| DATE: | | | | DAY OF WEEK: | | | | |
|---|---|---|---|---|---|---|---|---|
| TIME | | | | ORAL INTAKE | | | OUTPUT | |
| | am | pm | Caregiver | Medications / Supplements | Dosage amt. | Food | Liquid | Urine | BM |
| | | | | | | | | | |
| | | | | | | | | | |
| | | | | | | | | | |
| | | | | | | | | | |
| | | | | | | | | | |
| | | | | | | | | | |

Notes:

*"A soft answer turns off wrath, but a harsh word stirs up anger." Proverbs 15:1*

| HYGIENE Teeth/Bathe Hair/Nails | Physical Therapy | Occupational Therapy | Speech Therapy | Sleep | Vitals Y/N on chart | P/M Index |
|---|---|---|---|---|---|---|
| | | | | | | |
| | | | | | | |
| | | | | | | |
| | | | | | | |
| | | | | | | |
| | | | | | | |

Notes:

PAIN / MOOD
Index
0-10
0=none/good
10=high/angry

| DATE: | | | | DAY OF WEEK: | | | | | |
|---|---|---|---|---|---|---|---|---|---|
| TIME | | | | ORAL INTAKE | | | | OUTPUT | |
| | am | pm | Caregiver | Medications / Supplements | Dosage amt. | Food | Liquid | Urine | BM |
| | | | | | | | | | |
| | | | | | | | | | |
| | | | | | | | | | |
| | | | | | | | | | |
| | | | | | | | | | |
| | | | | | | | | | |

Notes:

*"Constant kindness can accomplish much. As the sun melts ice, kindness causes misunderstanding, mistrust, and hostility to evaporate."* Albert Schweitzer

| HYGIENE Teeth/Bathe Hair/Nails | Physical Therapy | Occupational Therapy | Speech Therapy | Sleep | Vitals Y/N on chart | P/M Index |
|---|---|---|---|---|---|---|
|  |  |  |  |  |  |  |
|  |  |  |  |  |  |  |
|  |  |  |  |  |  |  |
|  |  |  |  |  |  |  |
|  |  |  |  |  |  |  |
|  |  |  |  |  |  |  |

Notes:

PAIN / MOOD
Index
0-10
0=none/good
10=high/angry

| DATE: | | | | DAY OF WEEK: | | | | | |
|---|---|---|---|---|---|---|---|---|---|
| TIME | | | | ORAL INTAKE | | | | OUTPUT | |
| | am | pm | Caregiver | Medications / Supplements | Dosage amt. | Food | Liquid | Urine | BM |
| | | | | | | | | | |
| | | | | | | | | | |
| | | | | | | | | | |
| | | | | | | | | | |
| | | | | | | | | | |
| | | | | | | | | | |

Notes:

*"Want to snatch a day from the manacles of boredom? Do overgenerous deeds, acts beyond reimbursement, kindness without compensation. Do a deed for which you cannot be repaid."*
*Max Lucado*

| HYGIENE Teeth/Bathe Hair/Nails | Physical Therapy | Occupational Therapy | Speech Therapy | Sleep | Vitals Y/N on chart | P/M Index |
|---|---|---|---|---|---|---|
|  |  |  |  |  |  |  |
|  |  |  |  |  |  |  |
|  |  |  |  |  |  |  |
|  |  |  |  |  |  |  |
|  |  |  |  |  |  |  |
|  |  |  |  |  |  |  |

Notes:

PAIN / MOOD
Index
0-10
0=none/good
10=high/angry

| DATE: | | | | DAY OF WEEK: | | | | | |
|---|---|---|---|---|---|---|---|---|---|
| TIME | | | | ORAL INTAKE | | | | OUTPUT | |
| | am | pm | Caregiver | Medications / Supplements | Dosage amt. | Food | Liquid | Urine | BM |
| | | | | | | | | | |
| | | | | | | | | | |
| | | | | | | | | | |
| | | | | | | | | | |
| | | | | | | | | | |
| | | | | | | | | | |

Notes:

*"The greatest thing a person can do for the Heavenly Father is to be kind to some of His other children."* Henry Drummond

| HYGIENE Teeth/Bathe Hair/Nails | Physical Therapy | Occupational Therapy | Speech Therapy | Sleep | Vitals Y/N on chart | P/M Index |
|---|---|---|---|---|---|---|
|  |  |  |  |  |  |  |
|  |  |  |  |  |  |  |
|  |  |  |  |  |  |  |
|  |  |  |  |  |  |  |
|  |  |  |  |  |  |  |
|  |  |  |  |  |  |  |

Notes:

PAIN / MOOD
Index
0-10
0=none/good
10=high/angry

| DATE: | | | | DAY OF WEEK: | | | | | |
|---|---|---|---|---|---|---|---|---|---|
| TIME | | | | ORAL INTAKE | | | | OUTPUT | |
| | am | pm | Caregiver | Medications / Supplements | Dosage amt. | Food | Liquid | Urine | BM |
| | | | | | | | | | |
| | | | | | | | | | |
| | | | | | | | | | |
| | | | | | | | | | |
| | | | | | | | | | |
| | | | | | | | | | |

Notes:

*"At first they'll ask you WHY you are doing it. Later, they'll ask you HOW you did it."*
steadystrength.com

| HYGIENE Teeth/Bathe Hair/Nails | Physical Therapy | Occupational Therapy | Speech Therapy | Sleep | Vitals Y/N on chart | P/M Index |
|---|---|---|---|---|---|---|
|  |  |  |  |  |  |  |
|  |  |  |  |  |  |  |
|  |  |  |  |  |  |  |
|  |  |  |  |  |  |  |
|  |  |  |  |  |  |  |
|  |  |  |  |  |  |  |

Notes:

PAIN / MOOD
Index
0-10
0=none/good
10=high/angry

| DATE: | | | | DAY OF WEEK: | | | | | |
|---|---|---|---|---|---|---|---|---|---|
| TIME | | | | ORAL INTAKE | | | | OUTPUT | |
| | am | pm | Caregiver | Medications / Supplements | Dosage amt. | Food | Liquid | Urine | BM |
| | | | | | | | | | |
| | | | | | | | | | |
| | | | | | | | | | |
| | | | | | | | | | |
| | | | | | | | | | |
| | | | | | | | | | |

Notes:

*You'll have an opportunity to go out of your way to be kind to someone today. Don't let it slip by you.*

| HYGIENE Teeth/Bathe Hair/Nails | Physical Therapy | Occupational Therapy | Speech Therapy | Sleep | Vitals Y/N on chart | P/M Index |
|---|---|---|---|---|---|---|
|  |  |  |  |  |  |  |
|  |  |  |  |  |  |  |
|  |  |  |  |  |  |  |
|  |  |  |  |  |  |  |
|  |  |  |  |  |  |  |
|  |  |  |  |  |  |  |

Notes:

PAIN / MOOD
Index
0-10
0=none/good
10=high/angry

| DATE: | | | | DAY OF WEEK: | | | | | |
|---|---|---|---|---|---|---|---|---|---|
| TIME | | | | ORAL INTAKE | | | | OUTPUT | |
| | am | pm | Caregiver | Medications / Supplements | Dosage amt. | Food | Liquid | Urine | BM |
| | | | | | | | | | |
| | | | | | | | | | |
| | | | | | | | | | |
| | | | | | | | | | |
| | | | | | | | | | |
| | | | | | | | | | |

Notes:

*"Life is a succession of lessons which must be lived to be understood."*
Helen Keller, American Author and Activist

| HYGIENE Teeth/Bathe Hair/Nails | Physical Therapy | Occupational Therapy | Speech Therapy | Sleep | Vitals Y/N on chart | P/M Index |
|---|---|---|---|---|---|---|
|  |  |  |  |  |  |  |
|  |  |  |  |  |  |  |
|  |  |  |  |  |  |  |
|  |  |  |  |  |  |  |
|  |  |  |  |  |  |  |
|  |  |  |  |  |  |  |

Notes:

PAIN / MOOD
Index
0-10
0=none/good
10=high/angry

| DATE: | | | | DAY OF WEEK: | | | | |
|---|---|---|---|---|---|---|---|---|
| TIME | | | | ORAL INTAKE | | | | OUTPUT |
| | am | pm | Caregiver | Medications / Supplements | Dosage amt. | Food | Liquid | Urine | BM |
| | | | | | | | | | |
| | | | | | | | | | |
| | | | | | | | | | |
| | | | | | | | | | |
| | | | | | | | | | |
| | | | | | | | | | |

Notes:

*"Life is interesting. In the end, some of your greatest pains become your greatest strengths."*
*Drew Barrymore, American Actress*

| HYGIENE Teeth/Bathe Hair/Nails | Physical Therapy | Occupational Therapy | Speech Therapy | Sleep | Vitals Y/N on chart | P/M Index |
|---|---|---|---|---|---|---|
| | | | | | | |
| | | | | | | |
| | | | | | | |
| | | | | | | |
| | | | | | | |
| | | | | | | |

Notes:

PAIN / MOOD
Index
0-10
0=none/good
10=high/angry

| DATE: | | | | DAY OF WEEK: | | | | |
|---|---|---|---|---|---|---|---|---|
| TIME | | | | ORAL INTAKE | | | OUTPUT | |
| | am | pm | Caregiver | Medications / Supplements | Dosage amt. | Food | Liquid | Urine | BM |
| | | | | | | | | | |
| | | | | | | | | | |
| | | | | | | | | | |
| | | | | | | | | | |
| | | | | | | | | | |
| | | | | | | | | | |

Notes:

*"I have woven a parachute out of everything broken."* ~ William Stafford, American Poet

| HYGIENE Teeth/Bathe Hair/Nails | Physical Therapy | Occupational Therapy | Speech Therapy | Sleep | Vitals Y/N on chart | P/M Index |
|---|---|---|---|---|---|---|
|  |  |  |  |  |  |  |
|  |  |  |  |  |  |  |
|  |  |  |  |  |  |  |
|  |  |  |  |  |  |  |
|  |  |  |  |  |  |  |
|  |  |  |  |  |  |  |

Notes:

PAIN / MOOD
Index
0-10
0=none/good
10=high/angry

| DATE: | | | | DAY OF WEEK: | | | | |
|---|---|---|---|---|---|---|---|---|
| TIME | | | | ORAL INTAKE | | | OUTPUT | |
| | am | pm | Caregiver | Medications / Supplements | Dosage amt. | Food | Liquid | Urine | BM |
| | | | | | | | | | |
| | | | | | | | | | |
| | | | | | | | | | |
| | | | | | | | | | |
| | | | | | | | | | |
| | | | | | | | | | |

Notes:

*"The robbed that smiles, steals something from the thief."*
*~ William Shakespeare, English Poet and Playwright*

| HYGIENE Teeth/Bathe Hair/Nails | Physical Therapy | Occupational Therapy | Speech Therapy | Sleep | Vitals Y/N on chart | P/M Index |
|---|---|---|---|---|---|---|
| | | | | | | |
| | | | | | | |
| | | | | | | |
| | | | | | | |
| | | | | | | |
| | | | | | | |

Notes:

PAIN / MOOD
Index
0-10
0=none/good
10=high/angry

| DATE: | | | | DAY OF WEEK: | | | | |
|---|---|---|---|---|---|---|---|---|
| TIME | | | | ORAL INTAKE | | | OUTPUT | |
| | am | pm | Caregiver | Medications / Supplements | Dosage amt. | Food | Liquid | Urine | BM |
| | | | | | | | | | |
| | | | | | | | | | |
| | | | | | | | | | |
| | | | | | | | | | |
| | | | | | | | | | |
| | | | | | | | | | |

Notes:

*"Anxiety in a man's heart weighs him down, but a good word makes him glad."*
*~ Solomon, King of Israel; Proverbs 12:25*

| HYGIENE Teeth/Bathe Hair/Nails | Physical Therapy | Occupational Therapy | Speech Therapy | Sleep | Vitals Y/N on chart | P/M Index |
|---|---|---|---|---|---|---|
|  |  |  |  |  |  |  |
|  |  |  |  |  |  |  |
|  |  |  |  |  |  |  |
|  |  |  |  |  |  |  |
|  |  |  |  |  |  |  |
|  |  |  |  |  |  |  |

Notes:

PAIN / MOOD
Index
0-10
0=none/good
10=high/angry

| DATE: | | | | DAY OF WEEK: | | | | | |
|---|---|---|---|---|---|---|---|---|---|
| TIME | | | | ORAL INTAKE | | | | OUTPUT | |
| | am | pm | Caregiver | Medications / Supplements | Dosage amt. | Food | Liquid | Urine | BM |
| | | | | | | | | | |
| | | | | | | | | | |
| | | | | | | | | | |
| | | | | | | | | | |
| | | | | | | | | | |
| | | | | | | | | | |

Notes:

*"… fear not, for I am with you; be not dismayed, for I am your God; I will strengthen you, I will help you, I will uphold you with my righteous right hand." ~ Almighty God; Isaiah 41:10*

| HYGIENE Teeth/Bathe Hair/Nails | Physical Therapy | Occupational Therapy | Speech Therapy | Sleep | Vitals Y/N on chart | P/M Index |
|---|---|---|---|---|---|---|
|  |  |  |  |  |  |  |
|  |  |  |  |  |  |  |
|  |  |  |  |  |  |  |
|  |  |  |  |  |  |  |
|  |  |  |  |  |  |  |
|  |  |  |  |  |  |  |

Notes:

PAIN / MOOD
Index
0-10
0=none/good
10=high/angry

| DATE: | | | DAY OF WEEK: | | | | | |
|---|---|---|---|---|---|---|---|---|
| TIME | | | ORAL INTAKE | | | | OUTPUT | |
| | am | pm | Caregiver | Medications / Supplements | Dosage amt. | Food | Liquid | Urine | BM |
| | | | | | | | | | |
| | | | | | | | | | |
| | | | | | | | | | |
| | | | | | | | | | |
| | | | | | | | | | |
| | | | | | | | | | |

Notes:

*"Weeping may last for the night, but joy comes in the morning." Psalms 30:5*

| HYGIENE Teeth/Bathe Hair/Nails | Physical Therapy | Occupational Therapy | Speech Therapy | Sleep | Vitals Y/N on chart | P/M Index |
|---|---|---|---|---|---|---|
|  |  |  |  |  |  |  |
|  |  |  |  |  |  |  |
|  |  |  |  |  |  |  |
|  |  |  |  |  |  |  |
|  |  |  |  |  |  |  |
|  |  |  |  |  |  |  |

Notes:

PAIN / MOOD Index 0-10
0=none/good
10=high/angry

| DATE: | | | | DAY OF WEEK: | | | | |
|---|---|---|---|---|---|---|---|---|
| TIME | | | | ORAL INTAKE | | | OUTPUT | |
| | am | pm | Caregiver | Medications / Supplements | Dosage amt. | Food | Liquid | Urine | BM |
| | | | | | | | | | |
| | | | | | | | | | |
| | | | | | | | | | |
| | | | | | | | | | |
| | | | | | | | | | |
| | | | | | | | | | |

Notes:

*"We act as though comfort and luxury were the chief requirements of life, when all that we need to make us really happy is something to be enthusiastic about."* ~ Charles Kingsley

| HYGIENE Teeth/Bathe Hair/Nails | Physical Therapy | Occupational Therapy | Speech Therapy | Sleep | Vitals Y/N on chart | P/M Index |
|---|---|---|---|---|---|---|
| | | | | | | |
| | | | | | | |
| | | | | | | |
| | | | | | | |
| | | | | | | |
| | | | | | | |

Notes:

PAIN / MOOD
Index
0-10
0=none/good
10=high/angry

| DATE: | | | | DAY OF WEEK: | | | | | |
|---|---|---|---|---|---|---|---|---|---|
| TIME | | | | ORAL INTAKE | | | | OUTPUT | |
| | am | pm | Caregiver | Medications / Supplements | Dosage amt. | Food | Liquid | Urine | BM |
| | | | | | | | | | |
| | | | | | | | | | |
| | | | | | | | | | |
| | | | | | | | | | |
| | | | | | | | | | |
| | | | | | | | | | |

Notes:

*"Don't ever mistake my silence for ignorance, my calmness for acceptance, or my kindness for weakness."* www.quotesgram.com

| HYGIENE Teeth/Bathe Hair/Nails | Physical Therapy | Occupational Therapy | Speech Therapy | Sleep | Vitals Y/N on chart | P/M Index |
|---|---|---|---|---|---|---|
|  |  |  |  |  |  |  |
|  |  |  |  |  |  |  |
|  |  |  |  |  |  |  |
|  |  |  |  |  |  |  |
|  |  |  |  |  |  |  |
|  |  |  |  |  |  |  |

Notes:

PAIN / MOOD
Index
0-10
0=none/good
10=high/angry

| DATE: | | | | DAY OF WEEK: | | | | |
|---|---|---|---|---|---|---|---|---|
| TIME | | | | ORAL INTAKE | | | | OUTPUT |
| | am | pm | Caregiver | Medications / Supplements | Dosage amt. | Food | Liquid | Urine | BM |
| | | | | | | | | | |
| | | | | | | | | | |
| | | | | | | | | | |
| | | | | | | | | | |
| | | | | | | | | | |
| | | | | | | | | | |

**Notes:**

*"A little kindness from person to person is better than a vast love for all humankind."*
Richard Dehmel  QuotePixel.com

| HYGIENE Teeth/Bathe Hair/Nails | Physical Therapy | Occupational Therapy | Speech Therapy | Sleep | Vitals Y/N on chart | P/M Index |
|---|---|---|---|---|---|---|
| | | | | | | |
| | | | | | | |
| | | | | | | |
| | | | | | | |
| | | | | | | |
| | | | | | | |

Notes:

PAIN / MOOD
Index
0-10
0=none/good
10=high/angry

| DATE: | | | | DAY OF WEEK: | | | | | |
|---|---|---|---|---|---|---|---|---|---|
| TIME | | | | ORAL INTAKE | | | | OUTPUT | |
| | am | pm | Caregiver | Medications / Supplements | Dosage amt. | Food | Liquid | Urine | BM |
| | | | | | | | | | |
| | | | | | | | | | |
| | | | | | | | | | |
| | | | | | | | | | |
| | | | | | | | | | |
| | | | | | | | | | |

Notes:

*"Comparison is the thief of joy."* Teddy Roosevelt

| HYGIENE Teeth/Bathe Hair/Nails | Physical Therapy | Occupational Therapy | Speech Therapy | Sleep | Vitals Y/N on chart | P/M Index |
|---|---|---|---|---|---|---|
| | | | | | | |
| | | | | | | |
| | | | | | | |
| | | | | | | |
| | | | | | | |
| | | | | | | |

Notes:

PAIN / MOOD
Index
0-10
0=none/good
10=high/angry

| DATE: | | | | DAY OF WEEK: | | | | |
|---|---|---|---|---|---|---|---|---|
| TIME | | | | ORAL INTAKE | | | OUTPUT | |
| | am | pm | Caregiver | Medications / Supplements | Dosage amt. | Food | Liquid | Urine | BM |
| | | | | | | | | | |
| | | | | | | | | | |
| | | | | | | | | | |
| | | | | | | | | | |
| | | | | | | | | | |
| | | | | | | | | | |
| | | | | | | | | | |

Notes:

*"The only way to keep your health is to eat what you don't want, drink what you don't like, and do what you'd rather not."* Mark Twain

| HYGIENE Teeth/Bathe Hair/Nails | Physical Therapy | Occupational Therapy | Speech Therapy | Sleep | Vitals Y/N on chart | P/M Index |
|---|---|---|---|---|---|---|
| | | | | | | |
| | | | | | | |
| | | | | | | |
| | | | | | | |
| | | | | | | |
| | | | | | | |

Notes:

PAIN / MOOD Index
0-10
0=none/good
10=high/angry

| DATE: | | | | DAY OF WEEK: | | | | | |
|---|---|---|---|---|---|---|---|---|---|
| TIME | | | | ORAL INTAKE | | | | OUTPUT | |
| | am | pm | Caregiver | Medications / Supplements | Dosage amt. | Food | Liquid | Urine | BM |
| | | | | | | | | | |
| | | | | | | | | | |
| | | | | | | | | | |
| | | | | | | | | | |
| | | | | | | | | | |
| | | | | | | | | | |

Notes:

EAT well,
MOVE daily,
HYDRATE often,
SLEEP lots,
LOVE yourself & others,
Repeat for LIFE.

| HYGIENE Teeth/Bathe Hair/Nails | Physical Therapy | Occupational Therapy | Speech Therapy | Sleep | Vitals Y/N on chart | P/M Index |
|---|---|---|---|---|---|---|
| | | | | | | |
| | | | | | | |
| | | | | | | |
| | | | | | | |
| | | | | | | |
| | | | | | | |

Notes:

PAIN / MOOD
Index
0-10
0=none/good
10=high/angry

| DATE: | | | | DAY OF WEEK: | | | | |
|---|---|---|---|---|---|---|---|---|
| TIME | | | | ORAL INTAKE | | | OUTPUT | |
| | am | pm | Caregiver | Medications / Supplements | Dosage amt. | Food | Liquid | Urine | BM |
| | | | | | | | | | |
| | | | | | | | | | |
| | | | | | | | | | |
| | | | | | | | | | |
| | | | | | | | | | |
| | | | | | | | | | |

Notes:

*"You don't have to see the whole staircase, just take the FIRST STEP."*
aloeverancl.com

| HYGIENE Teeth/Bathe Hair/Nails | Physical Therapy | Occupational Therapy | Speech Therapy | Sleep | Vitals Y/N on chart | P/M Index |
|---|---|---|---|---|---|---|
|  |  |  |  |  |  |  |
|  |  |  |  |  |  |  |
|  |  |  |  |  |  |  |
|  |  |  |  |  |  |  |
|  |  |  |  |  |  |  |
|  |  |  |  |  |  |  |

Notes:

PAIN / MOOD
Index
0-10
0=none/good
10=high/angry

| DATE: | | | | DAY OF WEEK: | | | | | |
|---|---|---|---|---|---|---|---|---|---|
| TIME | | | | ORAL INTAKE | | | | OUTPUT | |
| | am | pm | Caregiver | Medications / Supplements | Dosage amt. | Food | Liquid | Urine | BM |
| | | | | | | | | | |
| | | | | | | | | | |
| | | | | | | | | | |
| | | | | | | | | | |
| | | | | | | | | | |
| | | | | | | | | | |

Notes:

*"Every accomplishment starts with the decision to try."* thequotepedia.com

| HYGIENE Teeth/Bathe Hair/Nails | Physical Therapy | Occupational Therapy | Speech Therapy | Sleep | Vitals Y/N on chart | P/M Index |
|---|---|---|---|---|---|---|
| | | | | | | |
| | | | | | | |
| | | | | | | |
| | | | | | | |
| | | | | | | |
| | | | | | | |

Notes:

PAIN / MOOD
Index
0-10
0=none/good
10=high/angry

| DATE: | | | | DAY OF WEEK: | | | | |
|---|---|---|---|---|---|---|---|---|
| TIME | | | | ORAL INTAKE | | | OUTPUT | |
| | am | pm | Caregiver | Medications / Supplements | Dosage amt. | Food | Liquid | Urine | BM |
| | | | | | | | | | |
| | | | | | | | | | |
| | | | | | | | | | |
| | | | | | | | | | |
| | | | | | | | | | |
| | | | | | | | | | |

Notes:

*"Happy is the person who finds wisdom, and the person who gains understanding."* Proverbs 3:13

| HYGIENE Teeth/Bathe Hair/Nails | Physical Therapy | Occupational Therapy | Speech Therapy | Sleep | Vitals Y/N on chart | P/M Index |
|---|---|---|---|---|---|---|
|  |  |  |  |  |  |  |
|  |  |  |  |  |  |  |
|  |  |  |  |  |  |  |
|  |  |  |  |  |  |  |
|  |  |  |  |  |  |  |
|  |  |  |  |  |  |  |

Notes:

PAIN / MOOD
Index
0-10
0=none/good
10=high/angry

| DATE: | | | | DAY OF WEEK: | | | | |
|---|---|---|---|---|---|---|---|---|
| TIME | | | | ORAL INTAKE | | | OUTPUT | |
| am | pm | Caregiver | Medications / Supplements | Dosage amt. | Food | Liquid | Urine | BM |
| | | | | | | | | |
| | | | | | | | | |
| | | | | | | | | |
| | | | | | | | | |
| | | | | | | | | |
| | | | | | | | | |

Notes:

*"The only time we have an excuse for looking down on a person is when we are helping lift them up."*
*Jesse Jackson*

| HYGIENE Teeth/Bathe Hair/Nails | Physical Therapy | Occupational Therapy | Speech Therapy | Sleep | Vitals Y/N on chart | P/M Index |
|---|---|---|---|---|---|---|
| | | | | | | |
| | | | | | | |
| | | | | | | |
| | | | | | | |
| | | | | | | |
| | | | | | | |

Notes:

PAIN / MOOD
Index
0-10
0=none/good
10=high/angry

| DATE: | | | | DAY OF WEEK: | | | | | |
|---|---|---|---|---|---|---|---|---|---|
| TIME | | | | ORAL INTAKE | | | | OUTPUT | |
| | am | pm | Caregiver | Medications / Supplements | Dosage amt. | Food | Liquid | Urine | BM |
| | | | | | | | | | |
| | | | | | | | | | |
| | | | | | | | | | |
| | | | | | | | | | |
| | | | | | | | | | |
| | | | | | | | | | |

Notes:

"God is our refuge and strength, a very present help in trouble." Psalm 46:1

| HYGIENE Teeth/Bathe Hair/Nails | Physical Therapy | Occupational Therapy | Speech Therapy | Sleep | Vitals Y/N on chart | P/M Index |
|---|---|---|---|---|---|---|
|  |  |  |  |  |  |  |
|  |  |  |  |  |  |  |
|  |  |  |  |  |  |  |
|  |  |  |  |  |  |  |
|  |  |  |  |  |  |  |
|  |  |  |  |  |  |  |

Notes:

PAIN / MOOD
Index
0-10
0=none/good
10=high/angry

| DATE: | | | | DAY OF WEEK: | | | | |
|---|---|---|---|---|---|---|---|---|
| TIME | | | | ORAL INTAKE | | | OUTPUT | |
| | am | pm | Caregiver | Medications / Supplements | Dosage amt. | Food | Liquid | Urine | BM |
| | | | | | | | | | |
| | | | | | | | | | |
| | | | | | | | | | |
| | | | | | | | | | |
| | | | | | | | | | |
| | | | | | | | | | |

Notes:

*"The LORD is good, a stronghold in the day of trouble; he knows those who take refuge in him."*
*Nahum 1:7*

| HYGIENE Teeth/Bathe Hair/Nails | Physical Therapy | Occupational Therapy | Speech Therapy | Sleep | Vitals Y/N on chart | P/M Index |
|---|---|---|---|---|---|---|
|  |  |  |  |  |  |  |
|  |  |  |  |  |  |  |
|  |  |  |  |  |  |  |
|  |  |  |  |  |  |  |
|  |  |  |  |  |  |  |
|  |  |  |  |  |  |  |

Notes:

PAIN / MOOD
Index
0-10
0=none/good
10=high/angry

| DATE: | | | DAY OF WEEK: | | | | | |
|---|---|---|---|---|---|---|---|---|
| TIME | | | | ORAL INTAKE | | | OUTPUT | |
| | am | pm | Caregiver | Medications / Supplements | Dosage amt. | Food | Liquid | Urine | BM |
| | | | | | | | | | |
| | | | | | | | | | |
| | | | | | | | | | |
| | | | | | | | | | |
| | | | | | | | | | |
| | | | | | | | | | |
| | | | | | | | | | |

Notes:

*"Kindness is loving people more than they deserve."* Joseph Jubert

| HYGIENE Teeth/Bathe Hair/Nails | Physical Therapy | Occupational Therapy | Speech Therapy | Sleep | Vitals Y/N on chart | P/M Index |
|---|---|---|---|---|---|---|
|  |  |  |  |  |  |  |
|  |  |  |  |  |  |  |
|  |  |  |  |  |  |  |
|  |  |  |  |  |  |  |
|  |  |  |  |  |  |  |
|  |  |  |  |  |  |  |

Notes:

PAIN / MOOD
Index
0-10
0=none/good
10=high/angry

| DATE: | | | | DAY OF WEEK: | | | | |
|---|---|---|---|---|---|---|---|---|
| TIME | | | | ORAL INTAKE | | | OUTPUT | |
| | am | pm | Caregiver | Medications / Supplements | Dosage amt. | Food | Liquid | Urine | BM |
| | | | | | | | | | |
| | | | | | | | | | |
| | | | | | | | | | |
| | | | | | | | | | |
| | | | | | | | | | |
| | | | | | | | | | |

Notes:

"If you look for truth, you may find comfort in the end; if you look for comfort you will not get either comfort or truth only soft soap and wishful thinking to begin, and in the end, despair."  ~C. S. Lewis

| HYGIENE Teeth/Bathe Hair/Nails | Physical Therapy | Occupational Therapy | Speech Therapy | Sleep | Vitals Y/N on chart | P/M Index |
|---|---|---|---|---|---|---|
|  |  |  |  |  |  |  |
|  |  |  |  |  |  |  |
|  |  |  |  |  |  |  |
|  |  |  |  |  |  |  |
|  |  |  |  |  |  |  |
|  |  |  |  |  |  |  |

Notes:

PAIN / MOOD
Index
0-10
0=none/good
10=high/angry

| DATE: | | | | DAY OF WEEK: | | | | | |
|---|---|---|---|---|---|---|---|---|---|
| TIME | | | | ORAL INTAKE | | | | OUTPUT | |
| | am | pm | Caregiver | Medications / Supplements | Dosage amt. | Food | Liquid | Urine | BM |
| | | | | | | | | | |
| | | | | | | | | | |
| | | | | | | | | | |
| | | | | | | | | | |
| | | | | | | | | | |
| | | | | | | | | | |

Notes:

*"Cast your burden on the LORD, and he will sustain you." Psalms 55:22*

| HYGIENE Teeth/Bathe Hair/Nails | Physical Therapy | Occupational Therapy | Speech Therapy | Sleep | Vitals Y/N on chart | P/M Index |
|---|---|---|---|---|---|---|
|  |  |  |  |  |  |  |
|  |  |  |  |  |  |  |
|  |  |  |  |  |  |  |
|  |  |  |  |  |  |  |
|  |  |  |  |  |  |  |
|  |  |  |  |  |  |  |

Notes:

PAIN / MOOD
Index
0-10
0=none/good
10=high/angry

| DATE: | | | | DAY OF WEEK: | | | | | |
|---|---|---|---|---|---|---|---|---|---|
| TIME | | | | ORAL INTAKE | | | | OUTPUT | |
| | am | pm | Caregiver | Medications / Supplements | Dosage amt. | Food | Liquid | Urine | BM |
| | | | | | | | | | |
| | | | | | | | | | |
| | | | | | | | | | |
| | | | | | | | | | |
| | | | | | | | | | |
| | | | | | | | | | |

Notes:

*"You never know when one kind word or one act of encouragement may change a life forever."*
quoesgram.com

| HYGIENE Teeth/Bathe Hair/Nails | Physical Therapy | Occupational Therapy | Speech Therapy | Sleep | Vitals Y/N on chart | P/M Index |
|---|---|---|---|---|---|---|
|  |  |  |  |  |  |  |
|  |  |  |  |  |  |  |
|  |  |  |  |  |  |  |
|  |  |  |  |  |  |  |
|  |  |  |  |  |  |  |
|  |  |  |  |  |  |  |

Notes:

PAIN / MOOD
Index
0-10
0=none/good
10=high/angry

| DATE: | | | | DAY OF WEEK: | | | | |
|---|---|---|---|---|---|---|---|---|
| TIME | | | | ORAL INTAKE | | | OUTPUT | |
| | am | pm | Caregiver | Medications / Supplements | Dosage amt. | Food | Liquid | Urine | BM |
| | | | | | | | | | |
| | | | | | | | | | |
| | | | | | | | | | |
| | | | | | | | | | |
| | | | | | | | | | |
| | | | | | | | | | |

Notes:

*"Love, joy, peace, patience, kindness, goodness, faithfulness, gentleness, and self-control. To these I commit my day."*

| HYGIENE Teeth/Bathe Hair/Nails | Physical Therapy | Occupational Therapy | Speech Therapy | Sleep | Vitals Y/N on chart | P/M Index |
|---|---|---|---|---|---|---|
| | | | | | | |
| | | | | | | |
| | | | | | | |
| | | | | | | |
| | | | | | | |
| | | | | | | |

Notes:

PAIN / MOOD
Index
0-10
0=none/good
10=high/angry

| DATE: | | | | DAY OF WEEK: | | | | | |
|---|---|---|---|---|---|---|---|---|---|
| TIME | | | | ORAL INTAKE | | | | OUTPUT | |
| | am | pm | Caregiver | Medications / Supplements | Dosage amt. | Food | Liquid | Urine | BM |
| | | | | | | | | | |
| | | | | | | | | | |
| | | | | | | | | | |
| | | | | | | | | | |
| | | | | | | | | | |
| | | | | | | | | | |

Notes:

*"When I get a headache, I follow the directions on the bottle. I TAKE TWO ASPIRIN and KEEP AWAY FROM CHILDREN."* clickypix.com

| HYGIENE Teeth/Bathe Hair/Nails | Physical Therapy | Occupational Therapy | Speech Therapy | Sleep | Vitals Y/N on chart | P/M Index |
|---|---|---|---|---|---|---|
|  |  |  |  |  |  |  |
|  |  |  |  |  |  |  |
|  |  |  |  |  |  |  |
|  |  |  |  |  |  |  |
|  |  |  |  |  |  |  |
|  |  |  |  |  |  |  |

Notes:

PAIN / MOOD
Index
0-10
0=none/good
10=high/angry

| DATE: | | | | DAY OF WEEK: | | | | |
|---|---|---|---|---|---|---|---|---|
| TIME | | | | ORAL INTAKE | | | OUTPUT | |
| | am | pm | Caregiver | Medications / Supplements | Dosage amt. | Food | Liquid | Urine | BM |
| | | | | | | | | | |
| | | | | | | | | | |
| | | | | | | | | | |
| | | | | | | | | | |
| | | | | | | | | | |
| | | | | | | | | | |

Notes:

*"Life isn't about waiting for the storm to pass; it's about learning to dance in the rain!"*

| HYGIENE Teeth/Bathe Hair/Nails | Physical Therapy | Occupational Therapy | Speech Therapy | Sleep | Vitals Y/N on chart | P/M Index |
|---|---|---|---|---|---|---|
| | | | | | | |
| | | | | | | |
| | | | | | | |
| | | | | | | |
| | | | | | | |
| | | | | | | |

Notes:

**PAIN / MOOD Index**
0-10
0=none/good
10=high/angry

| DATE: | | | DAY OF WEEK: | | | | | |
|---|---|---|---|---|---|---|---|---|
| TIME | | | ORAL INTAKE | | | | OUTPUT | |
| | am | pm | Caregiver | Medications / Supplements | Dosage amt. | Food | Liquid | Urine | BM |
| | | | | | | | | | |
| | | | | | | | | | |
| | | | | | | | | | |
| | | | | | | | | | |
| | | | | | | | | | |
| | | | | | | | | | |

Notes:

"The Lord himself will fight for you. Just stay calm." Exodus 14:14

| HYGIENE Teeth/Bathe Hair/Nails | Physical Therapy | Occupational Therapy | Speech Therapy | Sleep | Vitals Y/N on chart | P/M Index |
|---|---|---|---|---|---|---|
|  |  |  |  |  |  |  |
|  |  |  |  |  |  |  |
|  |  |  |  |  |  |  |
|  |  |  |  |  |  |  |
|  |  |  |  |  |  |  |
|  |  |  |  |  |  |  |

Notes:

PAIN / MOOD
Index
0-10
0=none/good
10=high/angry

| DATE: | | | | DAY OF WEEK: | | | | | |
|---|---|---|---|---|---|---|---|---|---|
| TIME | | | | ORAL INTAKE | | | | OUTPUT | |
| | am | pm | Caregiver | Medications / Supplements | Dosage amt. | Food | Liquid | Urine | BM |
| | | | | | | | | | |
| | | | | | | | | | |
| | | | | | | | | | |
| | | | | | | | | | |
| | | | | | | | | | |
| | | | | | | | | | |

**Notes:**

*"Inside me lives a skinny woman crying to get out. But I can usually shut her up with cookies."*
topsquote.blogspot.com

| HYGIENE Teeth/Bathe Hair/Nails | Physical Therapy | Occupational Therapy | Speech Therapy | Sleep | Vitals Y/N on chart | P/M Index |
|---|---|---|---|---|---|---|
| | | | | | | |
| | | | | | | |
| | | | | | | |
| | | | | | | |
| | | | | | | |
| | | | | | | |

Notes:

PAIN / MOOD
Index
0-10
0=none/good
10=high/angry

| DATE: | | | | DAY OF WEEK: | | | | |
|---|---|---|---|---|---|---|---|---|
| TIME | | | | ORAL INTAKE | | | | OUTPUT |
| | am | pm | Caregiver | Medications / Supplements | Dosage amt. | Food | Liquid | Urine | BM |
| | | | | | | | | | |
| | | | | | | | | | |
| | | | | | | | | | |
| | | | | | | | | | |
| | | | | | | | | | |
| | | | | | | | | | |

Notes:

*"So you have sorrow now, but I will see you again, and your hearts will rejoice, and no one will take your joy from you." - Jesus (John 16:22)*

| HYGIENE Teeth/Bathe Hair/Nails | Physical Therapy | Occupational Therapy | Speech Therapy | Sleep | Vitals Y/N on chart | P/M Index |
|---|---|---|---|---|---|---|
|  |  |  |  |  |  |  |
|  |  |  |  |  |  |  |
|  |  |  |  |  |  |  |
|  |  |  |  |  |  |  |
|  |  |  |  |  |  |  |
|  |  |  |  |  |  |  |

Notes:

PAIN / MOOD
Index
0-10
0=none/good
10=high/angry

DATE: DAY OF WEEK:

| TIME | | | | ORAL INTAKE | | | | OUTPUT | |
|---|---|---|---|---|---|---|---|---|---|
| | am | pm | Caregiver | Medications / Supplements | Dosage amt. | Food | Liquid | Urine | BM |
| | | | | | | | | | |
| | | | | | | | | | |
| | | | | | | | | | |
| | | | | | | | | | |
| | | | | | | | | | |
| | | | | | | | | | |

Notes:

*"You never know how STRONG you are until being strong is the ONLY choice you have."*
*funnypicblast.com*

| HYGIENE Teeth/Bathe Hair/Nails | Physical Therapy | Occupational Therapy | Speech Therapy | Sleep | Vitals Y/N on chart | P/M Index |
|---|---|---|---|---|---|---|
| | | | | | | |
| | | | | | | |
| | | | | | | |
| | | | | | | |
| | | | | | | |
| | | | | | | |

Notes:

PAIN / MOOD
Index
0-10
0=none/good
10=high/angry

| DATE: | | | DAY OF WEEK: | | | | | |
|---|---|---|---|---|---|---|---|---|
| TIME | | | | ORAL INTAKE | | | | OUTPUT |
| | am | pm | Caregiver | Medications / Supplements | Dosage amt. | Food | Liquid | Urine | BM |
| | | | | | | | | | |
| | | | | | | | | | |
| | | | | | | | | | |
| | | | | | | | | | |
| | | | | | | | | | |
| | | | | | | | | | |

Notes:

*The biggest lie I tell myself is 'I don't need to write that down. I'll remember it.'* bestofunworld.com

| HYGIENE Teeth/Bathe Hair/Nails | Physical Therapy | Occupational Therapy | Speech Therapy | Sleep | Vitals Y/N on chart | P/M Index |
|---|---|---|---|---|---|---|
| | | | | | | |
| | | | | | | |
| | | | | | | |
| | | | | | | |
| | | | | | | |
| | | | | | | |

Notes:

PAIN / MOOD
Index
0-10
0=none/good
10=high/angry

| DATE: | | | | DAY OF WEEK: | | | | |
|---|---|---|---|---|---|---|---|---|
| TIME | | | | ORAL INTAKE | | | OUTPUT | |
| | am | pm | Caregiver | Medications / Supplements | Dosage amt. | Food | Liquid | Urine | BM |
| | | | | | | | | | |
| | | | | | | | | | |
| | | | | | | | | | |
| | | | | | | | | | |
| | | | | | | | | | |
| | | | | | | | | | |

"True love never gives up. It cares more for others than for self. True love doesn't want what it doesn't have. Love doesn't strut or brag. It doesn't have a big head. True Love doesn't force itself on others. It doesn't have a 'me first' attitude. It doesn't fly off the handle. It doesn't keep score of the wrongs done to it. True love doesn't enjoy when others grovel, but it does take pleasure in the flowering of truth. True Love puts up with anything, trusts God always, always looks for the best, never looks back, but keeps going to the end. True Love never dies."

The Message (I Corinthians 13:4-8)

| HYGIENE Teeth/Bathe Hair/Nails | Physical Therapy | Occupational Therapy | Speech Therapy | Sleep | Vitals Y/N on chart | P/M Index |
|---|---|---|---|---|---|---|
|  |  |  |  |  |  |  |
|  |  |  |  |  |  |  |
|  |  |  |  |  |  |  |
|  |  |  |  |  |  |  |
|  |  |  |  |  |  |  |
|  |  |  |  |  |  |  |

Notes:

PAIN / MOOD
Index
0-10
0=none/good
10=high/angry

| DATE: | | | | DAY OF WEEK: | | | | |
|---|---|---|---|---|---|---|---|---|
| TIME | | | | ORAL INTAKE | | | | OUTPUT |
| | am | pm | Caregiver | Medications / Supplements | Dosage amt. | Food | Liquid | Urine | BM |
| | | | | | | | | | |
| | | | | | | | | | |
| | | | | | | | | | |
| | | | | | | | | | |
| | | | | | | | | | |
| | | | | | | | | | |

Notes:

*"Love and kindness are never wasted. They always make a difference. They bless the one who receives them, and bless you, the giver."* quotesgram.com

| HYGIENE Teeth/Bathe Hair/Nails | Physical Therapy | Occupational Therapy | Speech Therapy | Sleep | Vitals Y/N on chart | P/M Index |
|---|---|---|---|---|---|---|
|  |  |  |  |  |  |  |
|  |  |  |  |  |  |  |
|  |  |  |  |  |  |  |
|  |  |  |  |  |  |  |
|  |  |  |  |  |  |  |
|  |  |  |  |  |  |  |

Notes:

PAIN / MOOD
Index
0-10
0=none/good
10=high/angry

| DATE: | | | DAY OF WEEK: | | | | | |
|---|---|---|---|---|---|---|---|---|
| TIME | | | | ORAL INTAKE | | | | OUTPUT |
| | am | pm | Caregiver | Medications / Supplements | Dosage amt. | Food | Liquid | Urine | BM |
| | | | | | | | | | |
| | | | | | | | | | |
| | | | | | | | | | |
| | | | | | | | | | |
| | | | | | | | | | |
| | | | | | | | | | |

Notes:

*"God doesn't love us because we are good, but He makes us good because He loves us."*
*C. S. Lewis*

| HYGIENE Teeth/Bathe Hair/Nails | Physical Therapy | Occupational Therapy | Speech Therapy | Sleep | Vitals Y/N on chart | P/M Index |
|---|---|---|---|---|---|---|
| | | | | | | |
| | | | | | | |
| | | | | | | |
| | | | | | | |
| | | | | | | |
| | | | | | | |

Notes:

PAIN / MOOD
Index
0-10
0=none/good
10=high/angry

| DATE: | | | | DAY OF WEEK: | | | | | |
|---|---|---|---|---|---|---|---|---|---|
| TIME | | | | ORAL INTAKE | | | | OUTPUT | |
| | am | pm | Caregiver | Medications / Supplements | Dosage amt. | Food | Liquid | Urine | BM |
| | | | | | | | | | |
| | | | | | | | | | |
| | | | | | | | | | |
| | | | | | | | | | |
| | | | | | | | | | |
| | | | | | | | | | |

Notes:

*"Spread love wherever you go. Let no-one ever come to you without leaving happier."* Mother Teresa

| HYGIENE Teeth/Bathe Hair/Nails | Physical Therapy | Occupational Therapy | Speech Therapy | Sleep | Vitals Y/N on chart | P/M Index |
|---|---|---|---|---|---|---|
|  |  |  |  |  |  |  |
|  |  |  |  |  |  |  |
|  |  |  |  |  |  |  |
|  |  |  |  |  |  |  |
|  |  |  |  |  |  |  |
|  |  |  |  |  |  |  |

Notes:

PAIN / MOOD
Index
0-10
0=none/good
10=high/angry

| DATE: | | | | DAY OF WEEK: | | | | | |
|---|---|---|---|---|---|---|---|---|---|
| TIME | | | | ORAL INTAKE | | | | OUTPUT | |
| | am | pm | Caregiver | Medications / Supplements | Dosage amt. | Food | Liquid | Urine | BM |
| | | | | | | | | | |
| | | | | | | | | | |
| | | | | | | | | | |
| | | | | | | | | | |
| | | | | | | | | | |
| | | | | | | | | | |

Notes:

*"Thanks to God, not–only for 'rivers of endless joy above, but for 'streams of comfort here below." ~ Adoniram Judson*

| HYGIENE Teeth/Bathe Hair/Nails | Physical Therapy | Occupational Therapy | Speech Therapy | Sleep | Vitals Y/N on chart | P/M Index |
|---|---|---|---|---|---|---|
|  |  |  |  |  |  |  |
|  |  |  |  |  |  |  |
|  |  |  |  |  |  |  |
|  |  |  |  |  |  |  |
|  |  |  |  |  |  |  |
|  |  |  |  |  |  |  |

Notes:

PAIN / MOOD
Index
0-10
0=none/good
10=high/angry

| DATE: | | | DAY OF WEEK: | | | | | |
|---|---|---|---|---|---|---|---|---|
| TIME | | | | ORAL INTAKE | | | OUTPUT | |
| | am | pm | Caregiver | Medications / Supplements | Dosage amt. | Food | Liquid | Urine | BM |
| | | | | | | | | | |
| | | | | | | | | | |
| | | | | | | | | | |
| | | | | | | | | | |
| | | | | | | | | | |
| | | | | | | | | | |
| | | | | | | | | | |

Notes:

*"Seeing a spider isn't the biggest problem, it's when it disappears." curiano.com*

| HYGIENE Teeth/Bathe Hair/Nails | Physical Therapy | Occupational Therapy | Speech Therapy | Sleep | Vitals Y/N on chart | P/M Index |
|---|---|---|---|---|---|---|
|  |  |  |  |  |  |  |
|  |  |  |  |  |  |  |
|  |  |  |  |  |  |  |
|  |  |  |  |  |  |  |
|  |  |  |  |  |  |  |
|  |  |  |  |  |  |  |

Notes:

PAIN / MOOD
Index
0-10
0=none/good
10=high/angry

| DATE: | | | | DAY OF WEEK: | | | | | |
|---|---|---|---|---|---|---|---|---|---|
| TIME | | | | ORAL INTAKE | | | | OUTPUT | |
| | am | pm | Caregiver | Medications / Supplements | Dosage amt. | Food | Liquid | Urine | BM |
| | | | | | | | | | |
| | | | | | | | | | |
| | | | | | | | | | |
| | | | | | | | | | |
| | | | | | | | | | |
| | | | | | | | | | |

Notes:

*"Someone else is happy with less than what you have."* galeriesss.com

| HYGIENE Teeth/Bathe Hair/Nails | Physical Therapy | Occupational Therapy | Speech Therapy | Sleep | Vitals Y/N on chart | P/M Index |
|---|---|---|---|---|---|---|
| | | | | | | |
| | | | | | | |
| | | | | | | |
| | | | | | | |
| | | | | | | |
| | | | | | | |

Notes:

PAIN / MOOD
Index
0-10
0=none/good
10=high/angry

| DATE: | | | | DAY OF WEEK: | | | | |
|---|---|---|---|---|---|---|---|---|
| TIME | | | | ORAL INTAKE | | | | OUTPUT |
| | am | pm | Caregiver | Medications / Supplements | Dosage amt. | Food | Liquid | Urine | BM |
| | | | | | | | | | |
| | | | | | | | | | |
| | | | | | | | | | |
| | | | | | | | | | |
| | | | | | | | | | |
| | | | | | | | | | |

Notes:

*"When life hands you lemons, make grape juice; then sit back & watch as the world wonders how you did it." findmemes.com*

| HYGIENE Teeth/Bathe Hair/Nails | Physical Therapy | Occupational Therapy | Speech Therapy | Sleep | Vitals Y/N on chart | P/M Index |
|---|---|---|---|---|---|---|
|  |  |  |  |  |  |  |
|  |  |  |  |  |  |  |
|  |  |  |  |  |  |  |
|  |  |  |  |  |  |  |
|  |  |  |  |  |  |  |
|  |  |  |  |  |  |  |

Notes:

PAIN / MOOD
Index
0-10
0=none/good
10=high/angry

| DATE: | | | | DAY OF WEEK: | | | | |
|---|---|---|---|---|---|---|---|---|
| TIME | | | | ORAL INTAKE | | | OUTPUT | |
| am | pm | Caregiver | Medications / Supplements | Dosage amt. | Food | Liquid | Urine | BM |
| | | | | | | | | |
| | | | | | | | | |
| | | | | | | | | |
| | | | | | | | | |
| | | | | | | | | |
| | | | | | | | | |

**Notes:**

"People may be unkind, just be kind. They may cheat you, just be honest. They may criticize you, just be strong. They may forget your good deeds, just continue doing good because in the end, it's between you and God, not you and them." Author Unknown

| HYGIENE Teeth/Bathe Hair/Nails | Physical Therapy | Occupational Therapy | Speech Therapy | Sleep | Vitals Y/N on chart | P/M Index |
|---|---|---|---|---|---|---|
| | | | | | | |
| | | | | | | |
| | | | | | | |
| | | | | | | |
| | | | | | | |
| | | | | | | |

Notes:

PAIN / MOOD Index
0-10
0=none/good
10=high/angry

| DATE: | | | | DAY OF WEEK: | | | | | |
|---|---|---|---|---|---|---|---|---|---|
| TIME | | | | ORAL INTAKE | | | | OUTPUT | |
| | am | pm | Caregiver | Medications / Supplements | Dosage amt. | Food | Liquid | Urine | BM |
| | | | | | | | | | |
| | | | | | | | | | |
| | | | | | | | | | |
| | | | | | | | | | |
| | | | | | | | | | |
| | | | | | | | | | |

Notes:

*"I like when you smile, but I love it when I'm the reason!" findmemes.com*

| HYGIENE Teeth/Bathe Hair/Nails | Physical Therapy | Occupational Therapy | Speech Therapy | Sleep | Vitals Y/N on chart | P/M Index |
|---|---|---|---|---|---|---|
|  |  |  |  |  |  |  |
|  |  |  |  |  |  |  |
|  |  |  |  |  |  |  |
|  |  |  |  |  |  |  |
|  |  |  |  |  |  |  |
|  |  |  |  |  |  |  |

Notes:

PAIN / MOOD
Index
0-10
0=none/good
10=high/angry

| DATE: | | | | DAY OF WEEK: | | | | |
|---|---|---|---|---|---|---|---|---|
| TIME | | | | ORAL INTAKE | | | OUTPUT | |
| | am | pm | Caregiver | Medications / Supplements | Dosage amt. | Food | Liquid | Urine | BM |
| | | | | | | | | | |
| | | | | | | | | | |
| | | | | | | | | | |
| | | | | | | | | | |
| | | | | | | | | | |
| | | | | | | | | | |
| | | | | | | | | | |

Notes:

*"Be someone who makes someone else look forward to tomorrow."*

| HYGIENE Teeth/Bathe Hair/Nails | Physical Therapy | Occupational Therapy | Speech Therapy | Sleep | Vitals Y/N on chart | P/M Index |
|---|---|---|---|---|---|---|
| | | | | | | |
| | | | | | | |
| | | | | | | |
| | | | | | | |
| | | | | | | |
| | | | | | | |

Notes:

PAIN / MOOD
Index
0-10
0=none/good
10=high/angry

| DATE: | | | | DAY OF WEEK: | | | | | |
|---|---|---|---|---|---|---|---|---|---|
| TIME | | | | ORAL INTAKE | | | | OUTPUT | |
| | am | pm | Caregiver | Medications / Supplements | Dosage amt. | Food | Liquid | Urine | BM |
| | | | | | | | | | |
| | | | | | | | | | |
| | | | | | | | | | |
| | | | | | | | | | |
| | | | | | | | | | |
| | | | | | | | | | |
| | | | | | | | | | |

Notes:

*"Half our life is spent trying to find something to do with the time we have rushed through life trying to save."* Will Rogers

| HYGIENE Teeth/Bathe Hair/Nails | Physical Therapy | Occupational Therapy | Speech Therapy | Sleep | Vitals Y/N on chart | P/M Index |
|---|---|---|---|---|---|---|
| | | | | | | |
| | | | | | | |
| | | | | | | |
| | | | | | | |
| | | | | | | |
| | | | | | | |

Notes:

PAIN / MOOD
Index
0-10
0=none/good
10=high/angry

| DATE: | | | | DAY OF WEEK: | | | | | |
|---|---|---|---|---|---|---|---|---|---|
| TIME | | | | ORAL INTAKE | | | | OUTPUT | |
| | am | pm | Caregiver | Medications / Supplements | Dosage amt. | Food | Liquid | Urine | BM |
| | | | | | | | | | |
| | | | | | | | | | |
| | | | | | | | | | |
| | | | | | | | | | |
| | | | | | | | | | |
| | | | | | | | | | |

Notes:

*"Never let yesterday use up too much of today."* Will Rogers

| HYGIENE Teeth/Bathe Hair/Nails | Physical Therapy | Occupational Therapy | Speech Therapy | Sleep | Vitals Y/N on chart | P/M Index |
|---|---|---|---|---|---|---|
| | | | | | | |
| | | | | | | |
| | | | | | | |
| | | | | | | |
| | | | | | | |
| | | | | | | |

Notes:

PAIN / MOOD
Index
0-10
0=none/good
10=high/angry

| DATE: | | | | DAY OF WEEK: | | | | |
|---|---|---|---|---|---|---|---|---|
| TIME | | | | ORAL INTAKE | | | OUTPUT | |
| | am | pm | Caregiver | Medications / Supplements | Dosage amt. | Food | Liquid | Urine | BM |
| | | | | | | | | | |
| | | | | | | | | | |
| | | | | | | | | | |
| | | | | | | | | | |
| | | | | | | | | | |
| | | | | | | | | | |

Notes:

*"The worst thing that happens to you may be the best thing for you if you don't let it get the best of you."* Will Rogers

| HYGIENE Teeth/Bathe Hair/Nails | Physical Therapy | Occupational Therapy | Speech Therapy | Sleep | Vitals Y/N on chart | P/M Index |
|---|---|---|---|---|---|---|
|  |  |  |  |  |  |  |
|  |  |  |  |  |  |  |
|  |  |  |  |  |  |  |
|  |  |  |  |  |  |  |
|  |  |  |  |  |  |  |
|  |  |  |  |  |  |  |

Notes:

PAIN / MOOD
Index
0-10
0=none/good
10=high/angry

| DATE: | | | | DAY OF WEEK: | | | | |
|---|---|---|---|---|---|---|---|---|
| TIME | | | | ORAL INTAKE | | | OUTPUT | |
| | am | pm | Caregiver | Medications / Supplements | Dosage amt. | Food | Liquid | Urine | BM |
| | | | | | | | | | |
| | | | | | | | | | |
| | | | | | | | | | |
| | | | | | | | | | |
| | | | | | | | | | |
| | | | | | | | | | |

Notes:

*"Rumor travels faster, but it don't stay put as long as truth."* Will Rogers

| HYGIENE Teeth/Bathe Hair/Nails | Physical Therapy | Occupational Therapy | Speech Therapy | Sleep | Vitals Y/N on chart | P/M Index |
|---|---|---|---|---|---|---|
|  |  |  |  |  |  |  |
|  |  |  |  |  |  |  |
|  |  |  |  |  |  |  |
|  |  |  |  |  |  |  |
|  |  |  |  |  |  |  |
|  |  |  |  |  |  |  |

Notes:

PAIN / MOOD
Index
0-10
0=none/good
10=high/angry

| DATE: | | | | DAY OF WEEK: | | | | |
|---|---|---|---|---|---|---|---|---|
| TIME | | | | ORAL INTAKE | | | OUTPUT | |
| | am | pm | Caregiver | Medications / Supplements | Dosage amt. | Food | Liquid | Urine | BM |
| | | | | | | | | | |
| | | | | | | | | | |
| | | | | | | | | | |
| | | | | | | | | | |
| | | | | | | | | | |
| | | | | | | | | | |
| | | | | | | | | | |

Notes:

*"An ignorant person is one who doesn't know what you have just found out."* Will Rogers

| HYGIENE Teeth/Bathe Hair/Nails | Physical Therapy | Occupational Therapy | Speech Therapy | Sleep | Vitals Y/N on chart | P/M Index |
|---|---|---|---|---|---|---|
|  |  |  |  |  |  |  |
|  |  |  |  |  |  |  |
|  |  |  |  |  |  |  |
|  |  |  |  |  |  |  |
|  |  |  |  |  |  |  |
|  |  |  |  |  |  |  |

Notes:

PAIN / MOOD
Index
0-10
0=none/good
10=high/angry

| DATE: | | | | DAY OF WEEK: | | | | |
|---|---|---|---|---|---|---|---|---|
| TIME | | | | ORAL INTAKE | | | OUTPUT | |
| | am | pm | Caregiver | Medications / Supplements | Dosage amt. | Food | Liquid | Urine | BM |
| | | | | | | | | | |
| | | | | | | | | | |
| | | | | | | | | | |
| | | | | | | | | | |
| | | | | | | | | | |
| | | | | | | | | | |

Notes:

*"Good judgment comes from experience, and a lot of that comes from bad judgment."* Will Rogers

| HYGIENE Teeth/Bathe Hair/Nails | Physical Therapy | Occupational Therapy | Speech Therapy | Sleep | Vitals Y/N on chart | P/M Index |
|---|---|---|---|---|---|---|
| | | | | | | |
| | | | | | | |
| | | | | | | |
| | | | | | | |
| | | | | | | |
| | | | | | | |

Notes:

PAIN / MOOD
Index
0-10
0=none/good
10=high/angry

| DATE: | | | | DAY OF WEEK: | | | | | |
|---|---|---|---|---|---|---|---|---|---|
| TIME | | | | ORAL INTAKE | | | | OUTPUT | |
| | am | pm | Caregiver | Medications / Supplements | Dosage amt. | Food | Liquid | Urine | BM |
| | | | | | | | | | |
| | | | | | | | | | |
| | | | | | | | | | |
| | | | | | | | | | |
| | | | | | | | | | |
| | | | | | | | | | |
| | | | | | | | | | |

Notes:

*"Too many people spend money they haven't earned to buy things they don't want to impress people they don't like."* Will Rogers

| HYGIENE Teeth/Bathe Hair/Nails | Physical Therapy | Occupational Therapy | Speech Therapy | Sleep | Vitals Y/N on chart | P/M Index |
|---|---|---|---|---|---|---|
|  |  |  |  |  |  |  |
|  |  |  |  |  |  |  |
|  |  |  |  |  |  |  |
|  |  |  |  |  |  |  |
|  |  |  |  |  |  |  |
|  |  |  |  |  |  |  |

Notes:

PAIN / MOOD
Index
0-10
0=none/good
10=high/angry

| DATE: | | | | DAY OF WEEK: | | | | |
|---|---|---|---|---|---|---|---|---|
| TIME | | | | ORAL INTAKE | | | OUTPUT | |
| | am | pm | Caregiver | Medications / Supplements | Dosage amt. | Food | Liquid | Urine | BM |
| | | | | | | | | | |
| | | | | | | | | | |
| | | | | | | | | | |
| | | | | | | | | | |
| | | | | | | | | | |
| | | | | | | | | | |

Notes:

*"Live in such a way that you would not be ashamed to sell your parrot to the town gossip."*
Will Rogers

| HYGIENE Teeth/Bathe Hair/Nails | Physical Therapy | Occupational Therapy | Speech Therapy | Sleep | Vitals Y/N on chart | P/M Index |
|---|---|---|---|---|---|---|
| | | | | | | |
| | | | | | | |
| | | | | | | |
| | | | | | | |
| | | | | | | |
| | | | | | | |

Notes:

PAIN / MOOD
Index
0-10
0=none/good
10=high/angry

| DATE: | | | | DAY OF WEEK: | | | | |
|---|---|---|---|---|---|---|---|---|
| TIME | | | | ORAL INTAKE | | | OUTPUT | |
| | am | pm | Caregiver | Medications / Supplements | Dosage amt. | Food | Liquid | Urine | BM |
| | | | | | | | | | |
| | | | | | | | | | |
| | | | | | | | | | |
| | | | | | | | | | |
| | | | | | | | | | |
| | | | | | | | | | |

Notes:

*"The old believe everything, the middle-aged suspect everything, and the young know everything."*
Oscar Wilde

| HYGIENE Teeth/Bathe Hair/Nails | Physical Therapy | Occupational Therapy | Speech Therapy | Sleep | Vitals Y/N on chart | P/M Index |
|---|---|---|---|---|---|---|
|  |  |  |  |  |  |  |
|  |  |  |  |  |  |  |
|  |  |  |  |  |  |  |
|  |  |  |  |  |  |  |
|  |  |  |  |  |  |  |
|  |  |  |  |  |  |  |

Notes:

PAIN / MOOD
Index
0-10
0=none/good
10=high/angry

| DATE: | | | DAY OF WEEK: | | | | | |
|---|---|---|---|---|---|---|---|---|
| TIME | | | ORAL INTAKE | | | | OUTPUT | |
| am | pm | Caregiver | Medications / Supplements | Dosage amt. | Food | Liquid | Urine | BM |
| | | | | | | | | |
| | | | | | | | | |
| | | | | | | | | |
| | | | | | | | | |
| | | | | | | | | |
| | | | | | | | | |
| | | | | | | | | |

Notes:

*"Age is an issue of mind over matter. If you don't mind, it doesn't matter."* Mark Twain

| HYGIENE Teeth/Bathe Hair/Nails | Physical Therapy | Occupational Therapy | Speech Therapy | Sleep | Vitals Y/N on chart | P/M Index |
|---|---|---|---|---|---|---|
|  |  |  |  |  |  |  |
|  |  |  |  |  |  |  |
|  |  |  |  |  |  |  |
|  |  |  |  |  |  |  |
|  |  |  |  |  |  |  |
|  |  |  |  |  |  |  |

Notes:

PAIN / MOOD
Index
0-10
0=none/good
10=high/angry

| DATE: | | | | DAY OF WEEK: | | | | |
|---|---|---|---|---|---|---|---|---|
| TIME | | | | ORAL INTAKE | | | OUTPUT | |
| | am | pm | Caregiver | Medications / Supplements | Dosage amt. | Food | Liquid | Urine | BM |
| | | | | | | | | | |
| | | | | | | | | | |
| | | | | | | | | | |
| | | | | | | | | | |
| | | | | | | | | | |
| | | | | | | | | | |

Notes:

*"Anyone who stops learning is old, whether at twenty or eighty. Anyone who keeps learning stays young. The greatest thing in life is to keep your mind young." Henry Ford*

| HYGIENE Teeth/Bathe Hair/Nails | Physical Therapy | Occupational Therapy | Speech Therapy | Sleep | Vitals Y/N on chart | P/M Index |
|---|---|---|---|---|---|---|
|  |  |  |  |  |  |  |
|  |  |  |  |  |  |  |
|  |  |  |  |  |  |  |
|  |  |  |  |  |  |  |
|  |  |  |  |  |  |  |
|  |  |  |  |  |  |  |

Notes:

PAIN / MOOD Index
0-10
0=none/good
10=high/angry

| DATE: | | | | DAY OF WEEK: | | | | |
|---|---|---|---|---|---|---|---|---|
| TIME | | | | ORAL INTAKE | | | OUTPUT | |
| | am | pm | Caregiver | Medications / Supplements | Dosage amt. | Food | Liquid | Urine | BM |
| | | | | | | | | | |
| | | | | | | | | | |
| | | | | | | | | | |
| | | | | | | | | | |
| | | | | | | | | | |
| | | | | | | | | | |

Notes:

*"There is a fountain of youth: It is your mind, your talents, the creativity you bring to your life & the lives of people you love. When you learn to tap this source, you will have truly defeated age."*
Sophia Loren

| HYGIENE Teeth/Bathe Hair/Nails | Physical Therapy | Occupational Therapy | Speech Therapy | Sleep | Vitals Y/N on chart | P/M Index |
|---|---|---|---|---|---|---|
|  |  |  |  |  |  |  |
|  |  |  |  |  |  |  |
|  |  |  |  |  |  |  |
|  |  |  |  |  |  |  |
|  |  |  |  |  |  |  |
|  |  |  |  |  |  |  |

Notes:

PAIN / MOOD
Index
0-10
0=none/good
10=high/angry

| DATE: | | | | DAY OF WEEK: | | | | |
|---|---|---|---|---|---|---|---|---|
| TIME | | | | ORAL INTAKE | | | OUTPUT | |
| | am | pm | Caregiver | Medications / Supplements | Dosage amt. | Food | Liquid | Urine | BM |
| | | | | | | | | | |
| | | | | | | | | | |
| | | | | | | | | | |
| | | | | | | | | | |
| | | | | | | | | | |
| | | | | | | | | | |
| | | | | | | | | | |

Notes:

*"You can't help getting older, but you don't have to get old."* George Burns

| HYGIENE Teeth/Bathe Hair/Nails | Physical Therapy | Occupational Therapy | Speech Therapy | Sleep | Vitals Y/N on chart | P/M Index |
|---|---|---|---|---|---|---|
|  |  |  |  |  |  |  |
|  |  |  |  |  |  |  |
|  |  |  |  |  |  |  |
|  |  |  |  |  |  |  |
|  |  |  |  |  |  |  |
|  |  |  |  |  |  |  |

Notes:

PAIN / MOOD
Index
0-10
0=none/good
10=high/angry

| DATE: | | | | DAY OF WEEK: | | | | |
|---|---|---|---|---|---|---|---|---|
| TIME | | | | ORAL INTAKE | | | OUTPUT | |
| | am | pm | Caregiver | Medications / Supplements | Dosage amt. | Food | Liquid | Urine | BM |
| | | | | | | | | | |
| | | | | | | | | | |
| | | | | | | | | | |
| | | | | | | | | | |
| | | | | | | | | | |
| | | | | | | | | | |
| | | | | | | | | | |

Notes:

*"As I grow older, I pay less attention to what a person says. I just watch what they do."*
*Andrew Carnegie*

| HYGIENE Teeth/Bathe Hair/Nails | Physical Therapy | Occupational Therapy | Speech Therapy | Sleep | Vitals Y/N on chart | P/M Index |
|---|---|---|---|---|---|---|
| | | | | | | |
| | | | | | | |
| | | | | | | |
| | | | | | | |
| | | | | | | |
| | | | | | | |

Notes:

PAIN / MOOD
Index
0-10
0=none/good
10=high/angry

| DATE: | | | | DAY OF WEEK: | | | | |
|---|---|---|---|---|---|---|---|---|
| TIME | | | | ORAL INTAKE | | | OUTPUT | |
| | am | pm | Caregiver | Medications / Supplements | Dosage amt. | Food | Liquid | Urine | BM |
| | | | | | | | | | |
| | | | | | | | | | |
| | | | | | | | | | |
| | | | | | | | | | |
| | | | | | | | | | |
| | | | | | | | | | |

Notes:

*"The great secret, that all old people share, is that you really haven't changed in seventy or eighty years. Your body changes, but you don't change at all. And that, of course, causes great confusion."*
*Doris Lessing*

| HYGIENE Teeth/Bathe Hair/Nails | Physical Therapy | Occupational Therapy | Speech Therapy | Sleep | Vitals Y/N on chart | P/M Index |
|---|---|---|---|---|---|---|
|  |  |  |  |  |  |  |
|  |  |  |  |  |  |  |
|  |  |  |  |  |  |  |
|  |  |  |  |  |  |  |
|  |  |  |  |  |  |  |
|  |  |  |  |  |  |  |

Notes:

PAIN / MOOD
Index
0-10
0=none/good
10=high/angry

| DATE: | | | | DAY OF WEEK: | | | | |
|---|---|---|---|---|---|---|---|---|
| TIME | | | | ORAL INTAKE | | | OUTPUT | |
| | am | pm | Caregiver | Medications / Supplements | Dosage amt. | Food | Liquid | Urine | BM |
| | | | | | | | | | |
| | | | | | | | | | |
| | | | | | | | | | |
| | | | | | | | | | |
| | | | | | | | | | |
| | | | | | | | | | |

Notes:

*"Old minds are like old horses; you must exercise them if you wish to keep them in working order."*
*John Adams*

| HYGIENE Teeth/Bathe Hair/Nails | Physical Therapy | Occupational Therapy | Speech Therapy | Sleep | Vitals Y/N on chart | P/M Index |
|---|---|---|---|---|---|---|
|  |  |  |  |  |  |  |
|  |  |  |  |  |  |  |
|  |  |  |  |  |  |  |
|  |  |  |  |  |  |  |
|  |  |  |  |  |  |  |
|  |  |  |  |  |  |  |

Notes:

PAIN / MOOD Index
0-10
0=none/good
10=high/angry

| DATE: | | | | DAY OF WEEK: | | | | |
|---|---|---|---|---|---|---|---|---|
| TIME | | | | ORAL INTAKE | | | OUTPUT | |
| | am | pm | Caregiver | Medications / Supplements | Dosage amt. | Food | Liquid | Urine | BM |
| | | | | | | | | | |
| | | | | | | | | | |
| | | | | | | | | | |
| | | | | | | | | | |
| | | | | | | | | | |
| | | | | | | | | | |
| | | | | | | | | | |

Notes:

*"A diplomat is a man who always remembers a woman's birthday, but never remembers her age."*
*Robert Frost*

| HYGIENE Teeth/Bathe Hair/Nails | Physical Therapy | Occupational Therapy | Speech Therapy | Sleep | Vitals Y/N on chart | P/M Index |
|---|---|---|---|---|---|---|
| | | | | | | |
| | | | | | | |
| | | | | | | |
| | | | | | | |
| | | | | | | |
| | | | | | | |

Notes:

**PAIN / MOOD Index**
0-10
0=none/good
10=high/angry

| DATE: | | | | DAY OF WEEK: | | | | |
|---|---|---|---|---|---|---|---|---|
| TIME | | | | ORAL INTAKE | | | OUTPUT | |
| | am | pm | Caregiver | Medications / Supplements | Dosage amt. | Food | Liquid | Urine | BM |
| | | | | | | | | | |
| | | | | | | | | | |
| | | | | | | | | | |
| | | | | | | | | | |
| | | | | | | | | | |
| | | | | | | | | | |
| | | | | | | | | | |

Notes:

*"Men are like wine - some turn to vinegar, but the best improve with age."* Pope John XXIII

| HYGIENE Teeth/Bathe Hair/Nails | Physical Therapy | Occupational Therapy | Speech Therapy | Sleep | Vitals Y/N on chart | P/M Index |
|---|---|---|---|---|---|---|
|  |  |  |  |  |  |  |
|  |  |  |  |  |  |  |
|  |  |  |  |  |  |  |
|  |  |  |  |  |  |  |
|  |  |  |  |  |  |  |
|  |  |  |  |  |  |  |

Notes:

PAIN / MOOD
Index
0-10
0=none/good
10=high/angry

| DATE: | | | | DAY OF WEEK: | | | | |
|---|---|---|---|---|---|---|---|---|
| TIME | | | | ORAL INTAKE | | | OUTPUT | |
| | am | pm | Caregiver | Medications / Supplements | Dosage amt. | Food | Liquid | Urine | BM |
| | | | | | | | | | |
| | | | | | | | | | |
| | | | | | | | | | |
| | | | | | | | | | |
| | | | | | | | | | |
| | | | | | | | | | |

Notes:

*"Age appears to be best in four things: old wood best to burn, old wine to drink, old friends to trust, and old authors to read."* Francis Bacon

| HYGIENE Teeth/Bathe Hair/Nails | Physical Therapy | Occupational Therapy | Speech Therapy | Sleep | Vitals Y/N on chart | P/M Index |
|---|---|---|---|---|---|---|
| | | | | | | |
| | | | | | | |
| | | | | | | |
| | | | | | | |
| | | | | | | |
| | | | | | | |

Notes:

PAIN / MOOD
Index
0-10
0=none/good
10=high/angry

| DATE: | | | | DAY OF WEEK: | | | | |
|---|---|---|---|---|---|---|---|---|
| TIME | | | | ORAL INTAKE | | | OUTPUT | |
| | am | pm | Caregiver | Medications / Supplements | Dosage amt. | Food | Liquid | Urine | BM |
| | | | | | | | | | |
| | | | | | | | | | |
| | | | | | | | | | |
| | | | | | | | | | |
| | | | | | | | | | |
| | | | | | | | | | |
| | | | | | | | | | |

Notes:

*"Forty is the old age of youth; Fifty the youth of old age."* Victor Hugo

| HYGIENE Teeth/Bathe Hair/Nails | Physical Therapy | Occupational Therapy | Speech Therapy | Sleep | Vitals Y/N on chart | P/M Index |
|---|---|---|---|---|---|---|
|  |  |  |  |  |  |  |
|  |  |  |  |  |  |  |
|  |  |  |  |  |  |  |
|  |  |  |  |  |  |  |
|  |  |  |  |  |  |  |
|  |  |  |  |  |  |  |

Notes:

PAIN / MOOD
Index
0-10
0=none/good
10=high/angry

| DATE: | | | | DAY OF WEEK: | | | | | |
|---|---|---|---|---|---|---|---|---|---|
| TIME | | | | ORAL INTAKE | | | | OUTPUT | |
| | am | pm | Caregiver | Medications / Supplements | Dosage amt. | Food | Liquid | Urine | BM |
| | | | | | | | | | |
| | | | | | | | | | |
| | | | | | | | | | |
| | | | | | | | | | |
| | | | | | | | | | |
| | | | | | | | | | |
| | | | | | | | | | |

Notes:

*"Age is not important, unless you're a cheese."* Helen Hayes

| HYGIENE Teeth/Bathe Hair/Nails | Physical Therapy | Occupational Therapy | Speech Therapy | Sleep | Vitals Y/N on chart | P/M Index |
|---|---|---|---|---|---|---|
| | | | | | | |
| | | | | | | |
| | | | | | | |
| | | | | | | |
| | | | | | | |
| | | | | | | |

Notes:

PAIN / MOOD
Index
0-10
0=none/good
10=high/angry

| DATE: | | | | DAY OF WEEK: | | | | |
|---|---|---|---|---|---|---|---|---|
| TIME | | | | ORAL INTAKE | | | OUTPUT | |
| | am | pm | Caregiver | Medications / Supplements | Dosage amt. | Food | Liquid | Urine | BM |
| | | | | | | | | | |
| | | | | | | | | | |
| | | | | | | | | | |
| | | | | | | | | | |
| | | | | | | | | | |
| | | | | | | | | | |

Notes:

*"An archaeologist is the best husband a woman can have. The older she gets, the more interested he is in her."* Agatha Christie

| HYGIENE Teeth/Bathe Hair/Nails | Physical Therapy | Occupational Therapy | Speech Therapy | Sleep | Vitals Y/N on chart | P/M Index |
|---|---|---|---|---|---|---|
|  |  |  |  |  |  |  |
|  |  |  |  |  |  |  |
|  |  |  |  |  |  |  |
|  |  |  |  |  |  |  |
|  |  |  |  |  |  |  |
|  |  |  |  |  |  |  |

Notes:

PAIN / MOOD Index
0-10
0=none/good
10=high/angry

| DATE: | | | | DAY OF WEEK: | | | | |
|---|---|---|---|---|---|---|---|---|
| TIME | | | | ORAL INTAKE | | | OUTPUT | |
| | am | pm | Caregiver | Medications / Supplements | Dosage amt. | Food | Liquid | Urine | BM |
| | | | | | | | | | |
| | | | | | | | | | |
| | | | | | | | | | |
| | | | | | | | | | |
| | | | | | | | | | |
| | | | | | | | | | |
| | | | | | | | | | |

Notes:

*"Patience is bitter, but its fruit is sweet."* Jean-Jacques Rousseau

| HYGIENE Teeth/Bathe Hair/Nails | Physical Therapy | Occupational Therapy | Speech Therapy | Sleep | Vitals Y/N on chart | P/M Index |
|---|---|---|---|---|---|---|
| | | | | | | |
| | | | | | | |
| | | | | | | |
| | | | | | | |
| | | | | | | |
| | | | | | | |

Notes:

PAIN / MOOD
Index
0-10
0=none/good
10=high/angry

| DATE: | | | | DAY OF WEEK: | | | | |
|---|---|---|---|---|---|---|---|---|
| TIME | | | | ORAL INTAKE | | | OUTPUT | |
| | am | pm | Caregiver | Medications / Supplements | Dosage amt. | Food | Liquid | Urine | BM |
| | | | | | | | | | |
| | | | | | | | | | |
| | | | | | | | | | |
| | | | | | | | | | |
| | | | | | | | | | |
| | | | | | | | | | |
| | | | | | | | | | |

Notes:

*"Have patience. All things are difficult before they become easy."* Saadi

| HYGIENE Teeth/Bathe Hair/Nails | Physical Therapy | Occupational Therapy | Speech Therapy | Sleep | Vitals Y/N on chart | P/M Index |
|---|---|---|---|---|---|---|
|  |  |  |  |  |  |  |
|  |  |  |  |  |  |  |
|  |  |  |  |  |  |  |
|  |  |  |  |  |  |  |
|  |  |  |  |  |  |  |
|  |  |  |  |  |  |  |

Notes:

PAIN / MOOD
Index
0-10
0=none/good
10=high/angry

| DATE: | | | DAY OF WEEK: | | | | | |
|---|---|---|---|---|---|---|---|---|
| TIME | | | ORAL INTAKE | | | | OUTPUT | |
| am | pm | Caregiver | Medications / Supplements | Dosage amt. | Food | Liquid | Urine | BM |
| | | | | | | | | |
| | | | | | | | | |
| | | | | | | | | |
| | | | | | | | | |
| | | | | | | | | |
| | | | | | | | | |

Notes:

*"Even a happy life cannot be without a measure of darkness, and the word 'happy' would lose its meaning if it were not balanced by sadness. It is far better to take things as they come along with patience and equanimity."* Carl Jung

| HYGIENE Teeth/Bathe Hair/Nails | Physical Therapy | Occupational Therapy | Speech Therapy | Sleep | Vitals Y/N on chart | P/M Index |
|---|---|---|---|---|---|---|
| | | | | | | |
| | | | | | | |
| | | | | | | |
| | | | | | | |
| | | | | | | |
| | | | | | | |

Notes:

PAIN / MOOD Index
0-10
0=none/good
10=high/angry

| DATE: | | | | DAY OF WEEK: | | | | |
|---|---|---|---|---|---|---|---|---|
| TIME | | | | ORAL INTAKE | | | OUTPUT | |
| | am | pm | Caregiver | Medications / Supplements | Dosage amt. | Food | Liquid | Urine | BM |
| | | | | | | | | | |
| | | | | | | | | | |
| | | | | | | | | | |
| | | | | | | | | | |
| | | | | | | | | | |
| | | | | | | | | | |
| | | | | | | | | | |

Notes:

*"Patience and perseverance have a magical effect before which difficulties disappear and obstacles vanish."* John Quincy Adams

| HYGIENE Teeth/Bathe Hair/Nails | Physical Therapy | Occupational Therapy | Speech Therapy | Sleep | Vitals Y/N on chart | P/M Index |
|---|---|---|---|---|---|---|
|  |  |  |  |  |  |  |
|  |  |  |  |  |  |  |
|  |  |  |  |  |  |  |
|  |  |  |  |  |  |  |
|  |  |  |  |  |  |  |
|  |  |  |  |  |  |  |

Notes:

PAIN / MOOD
Index
0-10
0=none/good
10=high/angry

| DATE: | | | | DAY OF WEEK: | | | | | |
|---|---|---|---|---|---|---|---|---|---|
| TIME | | | | ORAL INTAKE | | | | OUTPUT | |
| | am | pm | Caregiver | Medications / Supplements | Dosage amt. | Food | Liquid | Urine | BM |
| | | | | | | | | | |
| | | | | | | | | | |
| | | | | | | | | | |
| | | | | | | | | | |
| | | | | | | | | | |
| | | | | | | | | | |

Notes:

*"Kindness doesn't cost a penny, but its value is beyond measure to the recipient."* Chris Holmes

| HYGIENE Teeth/Bathe Hair/Nails | Physical Therapy | Occupational Therapy | Speech Therapy | Sleep | Vitals Y/N on chart | P/M Index |
|---|---|---|---|---|---|---|
| | | | | | | |
| | | | | | | |
| | | | | | | |
| | | | | | | |
| | | | | | | |
| | | | | | | |

Notes:

PAIN / MOOD Index
0-10
0=none/good
10=high/angry

| DATE: | | | | DAY OF WEEK: | | | | |
|---|---|---|---|---|---|---|---|---|
| TIME | | | | ORAL INTAKE | | | OUTPUT | |
| | am | pm | Caregiver | Medications / Supplements | Dosage amt. | Food | Liquid | Urine | BM |
| | | | | | | | | | |
| | | | | | | | | | |
| | | | | | | | | | |
| | | | | | | | | | |
| | | | | | | | | | |
| | | | | | | | | | |

Notes:

*"It is easier to find men who will volunteer to die, than to find those who are willing to endure pain with patience."* Julius Caesar

| HYGIENE Teeth/Bathe Hair/Nails | Physical Therapy | Occupational Therapy | Speech Therapy | Sleep | Vitals Y/N on chart | P/M Index |
|---|---|---|---|---|---|---|
| | | | | | | |
| | | | | | | |
| | | | | | | |
| | | | | | | |
| | | | | | | |
| | | | | | | |

Notes:

PAIN / MOOD Index
0-10
0=none/good
10=high/angry

| DATE: | | | | DAY OF WEEK: | | | | |
|---|---|---|---|---|---|---|---|---|
| TIME | | | | ORAL INTAKE | | | OUTPUT | |
| | am | pm | Caregiver | Medications / Supplements | Dosage amt. | Food | Liquid | Urine | BM |
| | | | | | | | | | |
| | | | | | | | | | |
| | | | | | | | | | |
| | | | | | | | | | |
| | | | | | | | | | |
| | | | | | | | | | |

Notes:

*"Have patience with all things, but first of all with yourself."* St. Francis de Sales

| HYGIENE Teeth/Bathe Hair/Nails | Physical Therapy | Occupational Therapy | Speech Therapy | Sleep | Vitals Y/N on chart | P/M Index |
|---|---|---|---|---|---|---|
|  |  |  |  |  |  |  |
|  |  |  |  |  |  |  |
|  |  |  |  |  |  |  |
|  |  |  |  |  |  |  |
|  |  |  |  |  |  |  |
|  |  |  |  |  |  |  |

Notes:

PAIN / MOOD Index 0-10
0=none/good
10=high/angry

| DATE: | | | | DAY OF WEEK: | | | | |
|---|---|---|---|---|---|---|---|---|
| TIME | | | | ORAL INTAKE | | | OUTPUT | |
| | am | pm | Caregiver | Medications / Supplements | Dosage amt. | Food | Liquid | Urine | BM |
| | | | | | | | | | |
| | | | | | | | | | |
| | | | | | | | | | |
| | | | | | | | | | |
| | | | | | | | | | |
| | | | | | | | | | |
| | | | | | | | | | |

Notes:

*"The key to everything is patience. You get the chicken by hatching the egg, not by smashing it."*
*Arnold H. Glasgow*

| HYGIENE Teeth/Bathe Hair/Nails | Physical Therapy | Occupational Therapy | Speech Therapy | Sleep | Vitals Y/N on chart | P/M Index |
|---|---|---|---|---|---|---|
| | | | | | | |
| | | | | | | |
| | | | | | | |
| | | | | | | |
| | | | | | | |
| | | | | | | |

Notes:

PAIN / MOOD Index
0-10
0=none/good
10=high/angry

| DATE: | | | | DAY OF WEEK: | | | | |
|---|---|---|---|---|---|---|---|---|
| TIME | | | | ORAL INTAKE | | | OUTPUT | |
| | am | pm | Caregiver | Medications / Supplements | Dosage amt. | Food | Liquid | Urine | BM |
| | | | | | | | | | |
| | | | | | | | | | |
| | | | | | | | | | |
| | | | | | | | | | |
| | | | | | | | | | |
| | | | | | | | | | |

Notes:

*"Our real blessings often appear to us in the shape of pains, losses and disappointments; but let us have patience and we shall soon see them in their proper figures."* Joseph Addison

| HYGIENE Teeth/Bathe Hair/Nails | Physical Therapy | Occupational Therapy | Speech Therapy | Sleep | Vitals Y/N on chart | P/M Index |
|---|---|---|---|---|---|---|
| | | | | | | |
| | | | | | | |
| | | | | | | |
| | | | | | | |
| | | | | | | |
| | | | | | | |

Notes:

PAIN / MOOD
Index
0-10
0=none/good
10=high/angry

| DATE: | | | | DAY OF WEEK: | | | | |
|---|---|---|---|---|---|---|---|---|
| TIME | | | | ORAL INTAKE | | | OUTPUT | |
| | am | pm | Caregiver | Medications / Supplements | Dosage amt. | Food | Liquid | Urine | BM |
| | | | | | | | | | |
| | | | | | | | | | |
| | | | | | | | | | |
| | | | | | | | | | |
| | | | | | | | | | |
| | | | | | | | | | |
| | | | | | | | | | |

Notes:

*"For I know the plans I have for you," declares the Lord, "plans to prosper you and not to harm you, plans to give you hope & a future. Then you will call upon me & come & pray to me, and I will listen to you. You will seek me & find me when you seek me with all your heart. I will be found by you," declares the Lord. Jeremiah 29:11-14*

| HYGIENE
Teeth/Bathe
Hair/Nails | Physical
Therapy | Occupational
Therapy | Speech
Therapy | Sleep | Vitals
Y/N
on chart | P/M
Index |
|---|---|---|---|---|---|---|
|  |  |  |  |  |  |  |
|  |  |  |  |  |  |  |
|  |  |  |  |  |  |  |
|  |  |  |  |  |  |  |
|  |  |  |  |  |  |  |
|  |  |  |  |  |  |  |

Notes:

PAIN / MOOD
Index
0-10
0=none/good
10=high/angry

| DATE: | | | | DAY OF WEEK: | | | | |
|---|---|---|---|---|---|---|---|---|
| TIME | | | | ORAL INTAKE | | | OUTPUT | |
| | am | pm | Caregiver | Medications / Supplements | Dosage amt. | Food | Liquid | Urine | BM |
| | | | | | | | | | |
| | | | | | | | | | |
| | | | | | | | | | |
| | | | | | | | | | |
| | | | | | | | | | |
| | | | | | | | | | |

Notes:

*"No, I will be the pattern of all patience; I will say nothing."* William Shakespeare

| HYGIENE Teeth/Bathe Hair/Nails | Physical Therapy | Occupational Therapy | Speech Therapy | Sleep | Vitals Y/N on chart | P/M Index |
|---|---|---|---|---|---|---|
|  |  |  |  |  |  |  |
|  |  |  |  |  |  |  |
|  |  |  |  |  |  |  |
|  |  |  |  |  |  |  |
|  |  |  |  |  |  |  |
|  |  |  |  |  |  |  |

Notes:

PAIN / MOOD
Index
0-10
0=none/good
10=high/angry

| DATE: | | | | DAY OF WEEK: | | | | |
|---|---|---|---|---|---|---|---|---|
| TIME | | | | ORAL INTAKE | | | OUTPUT | |
| | am | pm | Caregiver | Medications / Supplements | Dosage amt. | Food | Liquid | Urine | BM |
| | | | | | | | | | |
| | | | | | | | | | |
| | | | | | | | | | |
| | | | | | | | | | |
| | | | | | | | | | |
| | | | | | | | | | |
| | | | | | | | | | |

Notes:

*"Patience is not simply the ability to wait - it's how we behave while we're waiting."* Joyce Meyer

| HYGIENE Teeth/Bathe Hair/Nails | Physical Therapy | Occupational Therapy | Speech Therapy | Sleep | Vitals Y/N on chart | P/M Index |
|---|---|---|---|---|---|---|
| | | | | | | |
| | | | | | | |
| | | | | | | |
| | | | | | | |
| | | | | | | |
| | | | | | | |

Notes:

PAIN / MOOD
Index
0-10
0=none/good
10=high/angry

# VITALS CHART

| Date | Temp | B/P | Pulse | Oxygen | Respir | Blood Glucose | Weight | Initials | NOTES: |
|------|------|-----|-------|--------|--------|---------------|--------|----------|--------|
|      |      |     |       |        |        |               |        |          |        |
|      |      |     |       |        |        |               |        |          |        |
|      |      |     |       |        |        |               |        |          |        |
|      |      |     |       |        |        |               |        |          |        |
|      |      |     |       |        |        |               |        |          |        |
|      |      |     |       |        |        |               |        |          |        |
|      |      |     |       |        |        |               |        |          |        |
|      |      |     |       |        |        |               |        |          |        |
|      |      |     |       |        |        |               |        |          |        |
|      |      |     |       |        |        |               |        |          |        |
|      |      |     |       |        |        |               |        |          |        |
|      |      |     |       |        |        |               |        |          |        |
|      |      |     |       |        |        |               |        |          |        |
|      |      |     |       |        |        |               |        |          |        |
|      |      |     |       |        |        |               |        |          |        |
|      |      |     |       |        |        |               |        |          |        |
|      |      |     |       |        |        |               |        |          |        |
|      |      |     |       |        |        |               |        |          |        |
|      |      |     |       |        |        |               |        |          |        |
|      |      |     |       |        |        |               |        |          |        |
|      |      |     |       |        |        |               |        |          |        |
|      |      |     |       |        |        |               |        |          |        |
|      |      |     |       |        |        |               |        |          |        |
|      |      |     |       |        |        |               |        |          |        |
|      |      |     |       |        |        |               |        |          |        |
|      |      |     |       |        |        |               |        |          |        |
|      |      |     |       |        |        |               |        |          |        |
|      |      |     |       |        |        |               |        |          |        |

Notes:

"Patience, persistence, & perspiration make an unbeatable combination for success." Napoleon Hill

| Date | VITALS | | | | | | | | NOTES: |
|---|---|---|---|---|---|---|---|---|---|
| | Temp | B/P | Pulse | Oxygen | Respir | Blood Glucose | Weight | Initials | |
| | | | | | | | | | |
| | | | | | | | | | |
| | | | | | | | | | |
| | | | | | | | | | |
| | | | | | | | | | |
| | | | | | | | | | |
| | | | | | | | | | |
| | | | | | | | | | |
| | | | | | | | | | |
| | | | | | | | | | |
| | | | | | | | | | |
| | | | | | | | | | |
| | | | | | | | | | |
| | | | | | | | | | |
| | | | | | | | | | |
| | | | | | | | | | |
| | | | | | | | | | |
| | | | | | | | | | |
| | | | | | | | | | |
| | | | | | | | | | |
| | | | | | | | | | |
| | | | | | | | | | |
| | | | | | | | | | |
| | | | | | | | | | |
| | | | | | | | | | |
| | | | | | | | | | |
| | | | | | | | | | |
| | | | | | | | | | |
| | | | | | | | | | |

Notes:

*"Take care of your body. It's the only place you have to live in."* Jim Rohn wishestrumpet.com

| Date | VITALS | | | | | | | NOTES: |
|---|---|---|---|---|---|---|---|---|
| | Temp | B/P | Pulse | Oxygen | Respir | Blood Glucose | Weight | Initials |
| | | | | | | | | |
| | | | | | | | | |
| | | | | | | | | |
| | | | | | | | | |
| | | | | | | | | |
| | | | | | | | | |
| | | | | | | | | |
| | | | | | | | | |
| | | | | | | | | |
| | | | | | | | | |
| | | | | | | | | |
| | | | | | | | | |
| | | | | | | | | |
| | | | | | | | | |
| | | | | | | | | |
| | | | | | | | | |
| | | | | | | | | |
| | | | | | | | | |
| | | | | | | | | |
| | | | | | | | | |
| | | | | | | | | |
| | | | | | | | | |
| | | | | | | | | |
| | | | | | | | | |
| | | | | | | | | |
| | | | | | | | | |
| | | | | | | | | |
| | | | | | | | | |
| | | | | | | | | |

Notes:

*"It is no coincidence that four of the letters in health are 'heal'."* Ed Northstrum

| Date | VITALS | | | | | | | | NOTES: |
| --- | --- | --- | --- | --- | --- | --- | --- | --- | --- |
| | Temp | B/P | Pulse | Oxygen | Respir | Blood Glucose | Weight | Initials | |
| | | | | | | | | | |
| | | | | | | | | | |
| | | | | | | | | | |
| | | | | | | | | | |
| | | | | | | | | | |
| | | | | | | | | | |
| | | | | | | | | | |
| | | | | | | | | | |
| | | | | | | | | | |
| | | | | | | | | | |
| | | | | | | | | | |
| | | | | | | | | | |
| | | | | | | | | | |
| | | | | | | | | | |
| | | | | | | | | | |
| | | | | | | | | | |
| | | | | | | | | | |
| | | | | | | | | | |
| | | | | | | | | | |
| | | | | | | | | | |
| | | | | | | | | | |
| | | | | | | | | | |
| | | | | | | | | | |
| | | | | | | | | | |
| | | | | | | | | | |
| | | | | | | | | | |
| | | | | | | | | | |
| | | | | | | | | | |
| | | | | | | | | | |

Notes:

*"Health is a relationship between you and your body. Nurture that relationship." K Delaporte*

| Date | **VITALS** | | | | | | | | NOTES: |
| | Temp | B/P | Pulse | Oxygen | Respir | Blood Glucose | Weight | Initials | |
|---|---|---|---|---|---|---|---|---|---|
| | | | | | | | | | |
| | | | | | | | | | |
| | | | | | | | | | |
| | | | | | | | | | |
| | | | | | | | | | |
| | | | | | | | | | |
| | | | | | | | | | |
| | | | | | | | | | |
| | | | | | | | | | |
| | | | | | | | | | |
| | | | | | | | | | |
| | | | | | | | | | |
| | | | | | | | | | |
| | | | | | | | | | |
| | | | | | | | | | |
| | | | | | | | | | |
| | | | | | | | | | |
| | | | | | | | | | |
| | | | | | | | | | |
| | | | | | | | | | |
| | | | | | | | | | |
| | | | | | | | | | |
| | | | | | | | | | |
| | | | | | | | | | |
| | | | | | | | | | |
| | | | | | | | | | |
| | | | | | | | | | |
| | | | | | | | | | |
| | | | | | | | | | |
| | | | | | | | | | |
| | | | | | | | | | |

*"If it doesn't challenge you, it doesn't change you."* quotesgram.com

| Date | VITALS | | | | | | | | NOTES: |
| --- | --- | --- | --- | --- | --- | --- | --- | --- | --- |
| | Temp | B/P | Pulse | Oxygen | Respir | Blood Glucose | Weight | Initials | |
| | | | | | | | | | |
| | | | | | | | | | |
| | | | | | | | | | |
| | | | | | | | | | |
| | | | | | | | | | |
| | | | | | | | | | |
| | | | | | | | | | |
| | | | | | | | | | |
| | | | | | | | | | |
| | | | | | | | | | |
| | | | | | | | | | |
| | | | | | | | | | |
| | | | | | | | | | |
| | | | | | | | | | |
| | | | | | | | | | |
| | | | | | | | | | |
| | | | | | | | | | |
| | | | | | | | | | |
| | | | | | | | | | |
| | | | | | | | | | |
| | | | | | | | | | |
| | | | | | | | | | |
| | | | | | | | | | |
| | | | | | | | | | |
| | | | | | | | | | |
| | | | | | | | | | |
| | | | | | | | | | |
| | | | | | | | | | |
| | | | | | | | | | |
| | | | | | | | | | |
| | | | | | | | | | |

*"Health is a great gift, contentment a great wealth, and faithfulness the best relationship." Buddha*

| Date | Temp | B/P | Pulse | Oxygen | Respir | Blood Glucose | Weight | Initials | NOTES: |
|------|------|-----|-------|--------|--------|---------------|--------|----------|--------|
|      |      |     |       |        |        |               |        |          |        |
|      |      |     |       |        |        |               |        |          |        |
|      |      |     |       |        |        |               |        |          |        |
|      |      |     |       |        |        |               |        |          |        |
|      |      |     |       |        |        |               |        |          |        |
|      |      |     |       |        |        |               |        |          |        |
|      |      |     |       |        |        |               |        |          |        |
|      |      |     |       |        |        |               |        |          |        |
|      |      |     |       |        |        |               |        |          |        |
|      |      |     |       |        |        |               |        |          |        |

(Columns under "VITALS": Temp, B/P, Pulse, Oxygen, Respir)

*"Hello, this is God. I will be handling all your problems and concerns today. That's my job. Your job is to give them to me, and then to trust me. Have a great day!" smileyme.com*

# ALTERNATIVE THERAPIES

**10 Ways to Love**
1. Listen without interrupting. (Proverbs 18)
2. Speak without accusing. (James 1:19)
3. Give without sparing. (Proverbs 21:26)
4. Pray without ceasing. (Colossians 1:9)
5. Answer without arguing. (Proverbs 17:1)
6. Share without pretending. (Ephesians 4:15)
7. Enjoy without complaint. (Philippians 2:14)
8. Trust without wavering. (I Corinthians 13:7)
9. Forgive without punishing. (Colossians 3:13)
10. Promise without forgetting. (Proverbs 13:12)

# FLUID BALANCE CHART

| Date | Time | INTAKE | | | | OUTPUT | | | | |
|------|------|--------|--|--|--|--------|--|--|--|--|
| | | Intravenous Fluid | Peg Parenteral Nutrition | Oral Intake | Cum Total | Vomit/Gastric Aspirate | Urine | Drains | Stoma | Cum Total |
| | | | | | | | | | | |
| | | | | | | | | | | |
| | | | | | | | | | | |
| | | | | | | | | | | |
| | | | | | | | | | | |
| | | | | | | | | | | |
| | | | | | | | | | | |
| | | | | | | | | | | |
| | | | | | | | | | | |
| | | | | | | | | | | |
| TOTALS | | | | | | | | | | |

**TOTAL INTAKE:**

**TOTAL OUTPUT:**

# FLUID BALANCE CHART

| | | INTAKE | | | | OUTPUT | | | | |
|---|---|---|---|---|---|---|---|---|---|---|
| Date | Time | Intravenous Fluid | Peg Parenteral Nutrition | Oral Intake | Cum Total | Vomit/Gastric Aspirate | Urine | Drains | Stoma | Cum Total |
| | | | | | | | | | | |
| | | | | | | | | | | |
| | | | | | | | | | | |
| | | | | | | | | | | |
| | | | | | | | | | | |
| | | | | | | | | | | |
| | | | | | | | | | | |
| | | | | | | | | | | |
| | | | | | | | | | | |
| | | | | | | | | | | |
| | | | | | | | | | | |
| | | | | | | | | | | |
| | | | | | | | | | | |
| | | | | | | | | | | |
| | | | | | | | | | | |
| | | | | | | | | | | |
| | | | | | | | | | | |
| | | | | | | | | | | |
| | | | | | | | | | | |
| | | | | | | | | | | |
| | | | | | | | | | | |
| | | | | | | | | | | |
| | | | | | | | | | | |
| | | | | | | | | | | |
| TOTALS | | | | | | | | | | |

**TOTAL INTAKE:**

**TOTAL OUTPUT:**

# FLUID BALANCE CHART

| Date | Time | INTAKE ||||| OUTPUT ||||
|---|---|---|---|---|---|---|---|---|---|
| | | Intravenous Fluid | Peg Parenteral Nutrition | Oral Intake | Cum Total | Vomit/Gastric Aspirate | Urine | Drains | Stoma | Cum Total |
| | | | | | | | | | | |
| **TOTALS** | | | | | | | | | | |

**TOTAL INTAKE:**

**TOTAL OUTPUT:**

# FLUID BALANCE CHART

| Date | Time | INTAKE ||||  OUTPUT ||||
|---|---|---|---|---|---|---|---|---|---|
| | | Intravenous Fluid | Peg Parenteral Nutrition | Oral Intake | Cum Total | Vomit/Gastric Aspirate | Urine | Drains | Stoma | Cum Total |
| | | | | | | | | | | |
| | | | | | | | | | | |
| | | | | | | | | | | |
| | | | | | | | | | | |
| | | | | | | | | | | |
| | | | | | | | | | | |
| | | | | | | | | | | |
| | | | | | | | | | | |
| | | | | | | | | | | |
| | | | | | | | | | | |
| | | | | | | | | | | |
| | | | | | | | | | | |
| | | | | | | | | | | |
| | | | | | | | | | | |
| | | | | | | | | | | |
| | | | | | | | | | | |
| | | | | | | | | | | |
| | | | | | | | | | | |
| | | | | | | | | | | |
| | | | | | | | | | | |
| | | | | | | | | | | |
| | | | | | | | | | | |
| | | | | | | | | | | |
| | | | | | | | | | | |
| | | | | | | | | | | |
| | | | | | | | | | | |
| | | | | | | | | | | |
| **TOTALS** | | | | | | | | | | |

**TOTAL INTAKE:**

**TOTAL OUTPUT:**

# FLUID BALANCE CHART

| | | INTAKE | | | | OUTPUT | | | | |
|---|---|---|---|---|---|---|---|---|---|---|
| Date | Time | Intravenous Fluid | Peg Parenteral Nutrition | Oral Intake | Cum Total | Vomit/Gastric Aspirate | Urine | Drains | Stoma | Cum Total |
| | | | | | | | | | | |
| | | | | | | | | | | |
| | | | | | | | | | | |
| | | | | | | | | | | |
| | | | | | | | | | | |
| | | | | | | | | | | |
| | | | | | | | | | | |
| | | | | | | | | | | |
| | | | | | | | | | | |
| | | | | | | | | | | |
| | | | | | | | | | | |
| | | | | | | | | | | |
| | | | | | | | | | | |
| | | | | | | | | | | |
| | | | | | | | | | | |
| | | | | | | | | | | |
| | | | | | | | | | | |
| | | | | | | | | | | |
| | | | | | | | | | | |
| | | | | | | | | | | |
| | | | | | | | | | | |
| | | | | | | | | | | |
| | TOTALS | | | | | | | | | |

**TOTAL INTAKE:**    **TOTAL OUTPUT:**

# CAREGIVER TIME SHEET

**CAREGIVER NAME:**

| YEAR | DATE | DAY OF WEEK | START TIME | END TIME | HOURS | TOTAL HOURS | NOTES: |
|------|------|-------------|------------|----------|-------|-------------|--------|
|      |      |             |            |          |       |             |        |
|      |      |             |            |          |       |             |        |
|      |      |             |            |          |       |             |        |
|      |      |             |            |          |       |             |        |
|      |      |             |            |          |       |             |        |
|      |      |             |            |          |       |             |        |
|      |      |             |            |          |       |             |        |
|      |      |             |            |          |       |             |        |
|      |      |             |            |          |       |             |        |
|      |      |             |            |          |       |             |        |
|      |      |             |            |          |       |             |        |
|      |      |             |            |          |       |             |        |
|      |      |             |            |          |       |             |        |
|      |      |             |            |          |       |             |        |
|      |      |             |            |          |       |             |        |
|      |      |             |            |          |       |             |        |
|      |      |             |            |          |       |             |        |
|      |      |             |            |          |       |             |        |
|      |      |             |            |          |       |             |        |
|      |      |             |            |          |       |             |        |
|      |      |             |            |          |       |             |        |
|      |      |             |            |          |       |             |        |
|      |      |             |            |          |       |             |        |
|      |      |             |            |          |       |             |        |
|      |      |             |            |          |       |             |        |
|      |      |             |            |          |       |             |        |
|      |      |             |            |          |       |             |        |
|      |      |             |            |          |       |             |        |
|      |      |             |            |          |       |             |        |
|      |      |             |            |          |       |             |        |
|      |      |             |            |          |       |             |        |

**CAREGIVER NAME:**                **CAREGIVER TIME SHEET**

# CAREGIVER TIME SHEET

**CAREGIVER NAME:**

| YEAR | DATE | DAY OF WEEK | START TIME | END TIME | HOURS | TOTAL HOURS | NOTES: |
|------|------|-------------|------------|----------|-------|-------------|--------|
|      |      |             |            |          |       |             |        |
|      |      |             |            |          |       |             |        |
|      |      |             |            |          |       |             |        |
|      |      |             |            |          |       |             |        |
|      |      |             |            |          |       |             |        |
|      |      |             |            |          |       |             |        |
|      |      |             |            |          |       |             |        |
|      |      |             |            |          |       |             |        |
|      |      |             |            |          |       |             |        |
|      |      |             |            |          |       |             |        |
|      |      |             |            |          |       |             |        |
|      |      |             |            |          |       |             |        |
|      |      |             |            |          |       |             |        |
|      |      |             |            |          |       |             |        |
|      |      |             |            |          |       |             |        |
|      |      |             |            |          |       |             |        |
|      |      |             |            |          |       |             |        |
|      |      |             |            |          |       |             |        |
|      |      |             |            |          |       |             |        |
|      |      |             |            |          |       |             |        |
|      |      |             |            |          |       |             |        |
|      |      |             |            |          |       |             |        |
|      |      |             |            |          |       |             |        |
|      |      |             |            |          |       |             |        |
|      |      |             |            |          |       |             |        |
|      |      |             |            |          |       |             |        |
|      |      |             |            |          |       |             |        |
|      |      |             |            |          |       |             |        |
|      |      |             |            |          |       |             |        |
|      |      |             |            |          |       |             |        |
|      |      |             |            |          |       |             |        |
|      |      |             |            |          |       |             |        |
|      |      |             |            |          |       |             |        |
|      |      |             |            |          |       |             |        |
|      |      |             |            |          |       |             |        |

**CAREGIVER NAME:**                              **CAREGIVER TIME SHEET**

# CAREGIVER TIME SHEET

**CAREGIVER NAME:**

| YEAR | DATE | DAY OF WEEK | START TIME | END TIME | HOURS | TOTAL HOURS | NOTES: |
|------|------|-------------|------------|----------|-------|-------------|--------|
|      |      |             |            |          |       |             |        |
|      |      |             |            |          |       |             |        |
|      |      |             |            |          |       |             |        |
|      |      |             |            |          |       |             |        |
|      |      |             |            |          |       |             |        |
|      |      |             |            |          |       |             |        |
|      |      |             |            |          |       |             |        |
|      |      |             |            |          |       |             |        |
|      |      |             |            |          |       |             |        |
|      |      |             |            |          |       |             |        |
|      |      |             |            |          |       |             |        |
|      |      |             |            |          |       |             |        |
|      |      |             |            |          |       |             |        |
|      |      |             |            |          |       |             |        |
|      |      |             |            |          |       |             |        |
|      |      |             |            |          |       |             |        |
|      |      |             |            |          |       |             |        |
|      |      |             |            |          |       |             |        |
|      |      |             |            |          |       |             |        |
|      |      |             |            |          |       |             |        |
|      |      |             |            |          |       |             |        |
|      |      |             |            |          |       |             |        |
|      |      |             |            |          |       |             |        |
|      |      |             |            |          |       |             |        |
|      |      |             |            |          |       |             |        |
|      |      |             |            |          |       |             |        |
|      |      |             |            |          |       |             |        |
|      |      |             |            |          |       |             |        |
|      |      |             |            |          |       |             |        |
|      |      |             |            |          |       |             |        |

**CAREGIVER TIME SHEET**

| CAREGIVER NAME: | | | | | | | CAREGIVER TIME SHEET |
|---|---|---|---|---|---|---|---|
| YEAR | DATE | DAY OF WEEK | START TIME | END TIME | HOURS | TOTAL HOURS | NOTES: |
| | | | | | | | |
| | | | | | | | |
| | | | | | | | |
| | | | | | | | |
| | | | | | | | |
| | | | | | | | |
| | | | | | | | |
| | | | | | | | |
| | | | | | | | |
| | | | | | | | |
| | | | | | | | |
| | | | | | | | |
| | | | | | | | |
| | | | | | | | |
| | | | | | | | |
| | | | | | | | |
| | | | | | | | |
| | | | | | | | |
| | | | | | | | |
| | | | | | | | |
| | | | | | | | |
| | | | | | | | |
| | | | | | | | |
| | | | | | | | |
| | | | | | | | |
| | | | | | | | |
| | | | | | | | |
| | | | | | | | |
| | | | | | | | |
| | | | | | | | |
| | | | | | | | |
| | | | | | | | |
| CAREGIVER NAME: | | | | | | | CAREGIVER TIME SHEET |

| CAREGIVER NAME: | | | | | | | CAREGIVER TIME SHEET |
|---|---|---|---|---|---|---|---|
| YEAR | DATE | DAY OF WEEK | START TIME | END TIME | HOURS | TOTAL HOURS | NOTES: |
| | | | | | | | |
| | | | | | | | |
| | | | | | | | |
| | | | | | | | |
| | | | | | | | |
| | | | | | | | |
| | | | | | | | |
| | | | | | | | |
| | | | | | | | |
| | | | | | | | |
| | | | | | | | |
| | | | | | | | |
| | | | | | | | |
| | | | | | | | |
| | | | | | | | |
| | | | | | | | |
| | | | | | | | |
| | | | | | | | |
| | | | | | | | |
| | | | | | | | |
| | | | | | | | |
| | | | | | | | |
| | | | | | | | |
| | | | | | | | |
| | | | | | | | |
| | | | | | | | |
| | | | | | | | |
| | | | | | | | |
| | | | | | | | |
| | | | | | | | |
| CAREGIVER NAME: | | | | | | | CAREGIVER TIME SHEET |

**CAREGIVER NAME:**                                            **CAREGIVER TIME SHEET**

| YEAR | DATE | DAY OF WEEK | START TIME | END TIME | HOURS | TOTAL HOURS | NOTES: |
|------|------|-------------|------------|----------|-------|-------------|--------|
|      |      |             |            |          |       |             |        |
|      |      |             |            |          |       |             |        |
|      |      |             |            |          |       |             |        |
|      |      |             |            |          |       |             |        |
|      |      |             |            |          |       |             |        |
|      |      |             |            |          |       |             |        |
|      |      |             |            |          |       |             |        |
|      |      |             |            |          |       |             |        |
|      |      |             |            |          |       |             |        |
|      |      |             |            |          |       |             |        |
|      |      |             |            |          |       |             |        |
|      |      |             |            |          |       |             |        |
|      |      |             |            |          |       |             |        |
|      |      |             |            |          |       |             |        |
|      |      |             |            |          |       |             |        |
|      |      |             |            |          |       |             |        |
|      |      |             |            |          |       |             |        |
|      |      |             |            |          |       |             |        |
|      |      |             |            |          |       |             |        |
|      |      |             |            |          |       |             |        |
|      |      |             |            |          |       |             |        |
|      |      |             |            |          |       |             |        |
|      |      |             |            |          |       |             |        |
|      |      |             |            |          |       |             |        |
|      |      |             |            |          |       |             |        |
|      |      |             |            |          |       |             |        |
|      |      |             |            |          |       |             |        |
|      |      |             |            |          |       |             |        |
|      |      |             |            |          |       |             |        |
|      |      |             |            |          |       |             |        |

**CAREGIVER NAME:**                                            **CAREGIVER TIME SHEET**

CAREGIVER NAME:    CAREGIVER TIME SHEET

| YEAR | DATE | DAY OF WEEK | START TIME | END TIME | HOURS | TOTAL HOURS | NOTES: |
|------|------|-------------|------------|----------|-------|-------------|--------|
|      |      |             |            |          |       |             |        |
|      |      |             |            |          |       |             |        |
|      |      |             |            |          |       |             |        |
|      |      |             |            |          |       |             |        |
|      |      |             |            |          |       |             |        |
|      |      |             |            |          |       |             |        |
|      |      |             |            |          |       |             |        |
|      |      |             |            |          |       |             |        |
|      |      |             |            |          |       |             |        |
|      |      |             |            |          |       |             |        |
|      |      |             |            |          |       |             |        |
|      |      |             |            |          |       |             |        |
|      |      |             |            |          |       |             |        |
|      |      |             |            |          |       |             |        |
|      |      |             |            |          |       |             |        |
|      |      |             |            |          |       |             |        |
|      |      |             |            |          |       |             |        |
|      |      |             |            |          |       |             |        |
|      |      |             |            |          |       |             |        |
|      |      |             |            |          |       |             |        |
|      |      |             |            |          |       |             |        |
|      |      |             |            |          |       |             |        |
|      |      |             |            |          |       |             |        |
|      |      |             |            |          |       |             |        |
|      |      |             |            |          |       |             |        |
|      |      |             |            |          |       |             |        |
|      |      |             |            |          |       |             |        |
|      |      |             |            |          |       |             |        |
|      |      |             |            |          |       |             |        |
|      |      |             |            |          |       |             |        |
| CAREGIVER NAME: |      |          |            |          |       | CAREGIVER TIME SHEET | |

**CAREGIVER NAME:**          **CAREGIVER TIME SHEET**

| YEAR | DATE | DAY OF WEEK | START TIME | END TIME | HOURS | TOTAL HOURS | NOTES: |
|---|---|---|---|---|---|---|---|
| | | | | | | | |
| | | | | | | | |
| | | | | | | | |
| | | | | | | | |
| | | | | | | | |
| | | | | | | | |
| | | | | | | | |
| | | | | | | | |
| | | | | | | | |
| | | | | | | | |
| | | | | | | | |
| | | | | | | | |
| | | | | | | | |
| | | | | | | | |
| | | | | | | | |
| | | | | | | | |
| | | | | | | | |
| | | | | | | | |
| | | | | | | | |
| | | | | | | | |
| | | | | | | | |
| | | | | | | | |
| | | | | | | | |
| | | | | | | | |
| | | | | | | | |
| | | | | | | | |
| | | | | | | | |
| | | | | | | | |
| | | | | | | | |
| | | | | | | | |
| | | | | | | | |

**CAREGIVER NAME:**          **CAREGIVER TIME SHEET**

| CAREGIVER NAME: | | | | | | | CAREGIVER TIME SHEET |
|---|---|---|---|---|---|---|---|
| YEAR | DATE | DAY OF WEEK | START TIME | END TIME | HOURS | TOTAL HOURS | NOTES: |
| | | | | | | | |
| | | | | | | | |
| | | | | | | | |
| | | | | | | | |
| | | | | | | | |
| | | | | | | | |
| | | | | | | | |
| | | | | | | | |
| | | | | | | | |
| | | | | | | | |
| | | | | | | | |
| | | | | | | | |
| | | | | | | | |
| | | | | | | | |
| | | | | | | | |
| | | | | | | | |
| | | | | | | | |
| | | | | | | | |
| | | | | | | | |
| | | | | | | | |
| | | | | | | | |
| | | | | | | | |
| | | | | | | | |
| | | | | | | | |
| | | | | | | | |
| | | | | | | | |
| | | | | | | | |
| | | | | | | | |
| | | | | | | | |
| | | | | | | | |
| CAREGIVER NAME: | | | | | | | CAREGIVER TIME SHEET |

| CAREGIVER NAME: | | | | | | | CAREGIVER TIME SHEET |
|---|---|---|---|---|---|---|---|
| YEAR | DATE | DAY OF WEEK | START TIME | END TIME | HOURS | TOTAL HOURS | NOTES: |
| | | | | | | | |
| | | | | | | | |
| | | | | | | | |
| | | | | | | | |
| | | | | | | | |
| | | | | | | | |
| | | | | | | | |
| | | | | | | | |
| | | | | | | | |
| | | | | | | | |
| | | | | | | | |
| | | | | | | | |
| | | | | | | | |
| | | | | | | | |
| | | | | | | | |
| | | | | | | | |
| | | | | | | | |
| | | | | | | | |
| | | | | | | | |
| | | | | | | | |
| | | | | | | | |
| | | | | | | | |
| | | | | | | | |
| | | | | | | | |
| | | | | | | | |
| | | | | | | | |
| | | | | | | | |
| | | | | | | | |
| | | | | | | | |
| | | | | | | | |
| CAREGIVER NAME: | | | | | | | CAREGIVER TIME SHEET |

CAREGIVER NAME:  CAREGIVER TIME SHEET

| YEAR | DATE | DAY OF WEEK | START TIME | END TIME | HOURS | TOTAL HOURS | NOTES: |
|---|---|---|---|---|---|---|---|
| | | | | | | | |

# CAREGIVER TIME SHEET

**CAREGIVER NAME:**

| YEAR | DATE | DAY OF WEEK | START TIME | END TIME | HOURS | TOTAL HOURS | NOTES: |
|------|------|-------------|------------|----------|-------|-------------|--------|
|      |      |             |            |          |       |             |        |
|      |      |             |            |          |       |             |        |
|      |      |             |            |          |       |             |        |
|      |      |             |            |          |       |             |        |
|      |      |             |            |          |       |             |        |
|      |      |             |            |          |       |             |        |
|      |      |             |            |          |       |             |        |
|      |      |             |            |          |       |             |        |
|      |      |             |            |          |       |             |        |
|      |      |             |            |          |       |             |        |
|      |      |             |            |          |       |             |        |
|      |      |             |            |          |       |             |        |
|      |      |             |            |          |       |             |        |
|      |      |             |            |          |       |             |        |
|      |      |             |            |          |       |             |        |
|      |      |             |            |          |       |             |        |
|      |      |             |            |          |       |             |        |
|      |      |             |            |          |       |             |        |
|      |      |             |            |          |       |             |        |
|      |      |             |            |          |       |             |        |
|      |      |             |            |          |       |             |        |
|      |      |             |            |          |       |             |        |
|      |      |             |            |          |       |             |        |
|      |      |             |            |          |       |             |        |
|      |      |             |            |          |       |             |        |
|      |      |             |            |          |       |             |        |
|      |      |             |            |          |       |             |        |
|      |      |             |            |          |       |             |        |
|      |      |             |            |          |       |             |        |
|      |      |             |            |          |       |             |        |
|      |      |             |            |          |       |             |        |
|      |      |             |            |          |       |             |        |

**CAREGIVER NAME:**  **CAREGIVER TIME SHEET**

| CAREGIVER NAME: | | | | | | | CAREGIVER TIME SHEET |
|---|---|---|---|---|---|---|---|
| YEAR | DATE | DAY OF WEEK | START TIME | END TIME | HOURS | TOTAL HOURS | NOTES: |
| | | | | | | | |
| | | | | | | | |
| | | | | | | | |
| | | | | | | | |
| | | | | | | | |
| | | | | | | | |
| | | | | | | | |
| | | | | | | | |
| | | | | | | | |
| | | | | | | | |
| | | | | | | | |
| | | | | | | | |
| | | | | | | | |
| | | | | | | | |
| | | | | | | | |
| | | | | | | | |
| | | | | | | | |
| | | | | | | | |
| | | | | | | | |
| | | | | | | | |
| | | | | | | | |
| | | | | | | | |
| | | | | | | | |
| | | | | | | | |
| | | | | | | | |
| | | | | | | | |
| | | | | | | | |
| | | | | | | | |
| | | | | | | | |
| | | | | | | | |
| | | | | | | | |
| | | | | | | | |
| | | | | | | | |
| CAREGIVER NAME: | | | | | | | CAREGIVER TIME SHEET |

# CAREGIVER TIME SHEET

**CAREGIVER NAME:**

| YEAR | DATE | DAY OF WEEK | START TIME | END TIME | HOURS | TOTAL HOURS | NOTES: |
|------|------|-------------|------------|----------|-------|-------------|--------|
|      |      |             |            |          |       |             |        |
|      |      |             |            |          |       |             |        |
|      |      |             |            |          |       |             |        |
|      |      |             |            |          |       |             |        |
|      |      |             |            |          |       |             |        |
|      |      |             |            |          |       |             |        |
|      |      |             |            |          |       |             |        |
|      |      |             |            |          |       |             |        |
|      |      |             |            |          |       |             |        |
|      |      |             |            |          |       |             |        |
|      |      |             |            |          |       |             |        |
|      |      |             |            |          |       |             |        |
|      |      |             |            |          |       |             |        |
|      |      |             |            |          |       |             |        |
|      |      |             |            |          |       |             |        |
|      |      |             |            |          |       |             |        |
|      |      |             |            |          |       |             |        |
|      |      |             |            |          |       |             |        |
|      |      |             |            |          |       |             |        |
|      |      |             |            |          |       |             |        |
|      |      |             |            |          |       |             |        |
|      |      |             |            |          |       |             |        |
|      |      |             |            |          |       |             |        |
|      |      |             |            |          |       |             |        |
|      |      |             |            |          |       |             |        |
|      |      |             |            |          |       |             |        |
|      |      |             |            |          |       |             |        |
|      |      |             |            |          |       |             |        |
|      |      |             |            |          |       |             |        |
|      |      |             |            |          |       |             |        |
|      |      |             |            |          |       |             |        |
|      |      |             |            |          |       |             |        |
|      |      |             |            |          |       |             |        |

**CAREGIVER NAME:**            **CAREGIVER TIME SHEET**

# HOSPITAL STAYS

(This is not intended to be a medical record, only a quick reference list to remind of recent hospital stays. For more information, please review actual medical records & discharge papers.)

| HOSPITAL | FROM | TO | REASON FOR ADMITTANCE | HOSPITALISTS | NOTES |
|---|---|---|---|---|---|
| | | | | | |
| | | | | | |
| | | | | | |
| | | | | | |
| | | | | | |
| | | | | | |
| | | | | | |

# DOCTOR VISITS

(This is not intended to be a medical record, only a quick reference list to remind of recent doctor appointments. For more information, please review actual medical records.)

| DOCTOR | DATE | SYMPTOMS | DIAGNOSIS | RECOMMENDATIONS | PRESCRIPTIONS/ PRESCIPTION CHANGES |
|---|---|---|---|---|---|
|  |  |  |  |  |  |
|  |  |  |  |  |  |
|  |  |  |  |  |  |
|  |  |  |  |  |  |
|  |  |  |  |  |  |
|  |  |  |  |  |  |
|  |  |  |  |  |  |

# QUESTIONS TO ASK DOCTOR
(For next phone call or Doctor Appointment)

| Customizable Chart | | | | |
|---|---|---|---|---|
| TITLE: | | | | |
|  |  |  |  |  |
|  |  |  |  |  |
|  |  |  |  |  |
|  |  |  |  |  |
|  |  |  |  |  |
|  |  |  |  |  |
|  |  |  |  |  |
|  |  |  |  |  |
|  |  |  |  |  |
|  |  |  |  |  |
|  |  |  |  |  |

CUSTOMIZABLE CHART

TITLE:

Extra Notes:

Extra Notes:

Made in the USA
Middletown, DE
08 January 2019